Procreative Responsibility and Assisted Reproductive Technologies

This book rethinks procreative responsibility considering the continuous development of Assisted Reproductive Technologies. It presents a person-affecting moral argument, highlighting that the potential availability of future Assisted Reproductive Technologies brings out new procreative obligations.

Traditionally, Assisted Reproductive Technologies are understood as practices aimed at extending the procreative freedom of prospective parents. However, some scholars argue that they also give rise to new moral constraints. This book builds on this viewpoint by presenting a person-affecting perspective on the impact of current and future Assisted Reproductive Technologies on procreative responsibility, with a specific focus on reproductive Genome Editing and ectogenesis. The author shows that this perspective is defensible both from a consequences-based person-affecting perspective and from a person-affecting account that considers morally relevant intuitions and attitudes.

Procreative Responsibility and Assisted Reproductive Technologies will appeal to scholars and advanced students working in bioethics and procreative ethics.

Davide Battisti is a postdoctoral researcher in Philosophy of Law and Bioethics at the Department of Law of the University of Bergamo. He also serves as an adjunct professor of Bioethics in the Politics, Philosophy, and Public Affairs Program at the University of Milan and the Vita-Salute San Raffaele University. He has published several papers on topics such as reproductive ethics, the allocation of scarce healthcare resources, the ethics of science communication, and research ethics. His work has appeared in journals such as *Bioethics*, the *Journal of Medical Ethics*, *Social Epistemology*, and *Ethics of Human Research*.

Routledge Research in Applied Ethics

For more information about this series, please visit: https://www.routledge.com/Routledge-Research-in-Applied-Ethics/book-series/RRAES

Procreative Responsibility and Assisted Reproductive Technologies

Davide Battisti

Routledge
Taylor & Francis Group

NEW YORK AND LONDON

First published 2025
by Routledge
605 Third Avenue, New York, NY 10158

and by Routledge
4 Park Square, Milton Park, Abingdon, Oxon, OX14 4RN

Routledge is an imprint of the Taylor & Francis Group, an informa business

© 2025 Davide Battisti

Library of Congress Cataloging-in-Publication Data
Names: Battisti, Davide, author.
Title: Procreative responsibility and assisted reproductive technologies / Davide Battisti.
Description: New York, NY : Routledge, 2024. | Series: Routledge research in applied ethics | Includes bibliographical references and index.
Identifiers: LCCN 2024007156 (print) | LCCN 2024007157 (ebook) | ISBN 9781032652085 (hardback) | ISBN 9781032654690 (paperback) | ISBN 9781032654683 (ebook)
Subjects: LCSH: Reproductive technology—Moral and ethical aspects.
Classification: LCC RG133.5 .B375 2024 (print) | LCC RG133.5 (ebook) | DDC 618.1/78—dc23/eng/20240411
LC record available at https://lccn.loc.gov/2024007156
LC ebook record available at https://lccn.loc.gov/2024007157

ISBN: 978-1-032-65208-5 (hbk)
ISBN: 978-1-032-65469-0 (pbk)
ISBN: 978-1-032-65468-3 (ebk)

DOI: 10.4324/9781032654683

Typeset in Sabon
by codeMantra

Contents

Introduction

In ancient Egypt, people already had methods for determining whether a person was pregnant and whether the fetus in the womb was male or female. An often-mentioned procedure involved pouring the pregnant person's urine onto barley and wheat grains. If the grains sprouted, this indicated that the person was pregnant; if the barley germinated first, it was established that the unborn child would be a boy (Haimov-Kochman et al., 2005). Similarly, in 14th-century China, a method was formulated to predict the sex of a baby based on the month of conception and the mother's age; a similar calendar was also used by the Maya civilization (Klipstein, 2017). Following the discovery of sperm in 1677, scientists believed they could predict an offspring's appearance using a microscope (Klipstein, 2017).

These are just some historical examples demonstrating how human beings have always sought information on human reproduction and, therefore, attempted to influence it. The scientific advancements of recent decades have provided far more effective tools than those described above to satisfy this inherent human inclination. As detailed in Chapter 1, it is now possible to identify congenital diseases in a fetus through prenatal genetic testing, providing prospective parents with crucial information that could decisively guide their choices. Increasingly, couples experiencing fertility issues can turn to *In Vitro* Fertilization (IVF), thereby maximizing their chances of realizing their dream of becoming parents. Furthermore, IVF provides access to multiple embryos, from which detailed information can be obtained through preimplantation genetic testing. Such a procedure enables prospective parents to select embryos based on specific traits, such as the likelihood of developing certain genetic diseases or the sex of the child.

Although these technologies are strictly regulated in several countries, there is no doubt that they offer people with the opportunity and desire to use them a wider range of procreative choices than in the past. It is not surprising that, in the contemporary context, Assisted

DOI: 10.4324/9781032654683-1

Reproductive Technologies (ARTs) are commonly considered tools that extend prospective parents' control over certain aspects of procreation and, consequently, their ability to determine progeny, increasing their procreative freedom. This becomes even more evident considering that ARTs are constantly improving and offer increasing efficacy and safety rates. Furthermore, ongoing developments in genetics allow for the identification of more and more genetic conditions (not only pathological), and such information could, at least in principle, more informatively guide procreative choices and preferences.

In the future, it will not only be possible to select which early embryos to transfer into the womb, but it might also be feasible to modify them to prevent genetic diseases or even enhance certain non-pathological traits of the future child through reproductive Genome Editing (rGE). We are already approaching such a milestone, as highlighted by a 2018 *New York Times* headline "Once Science Fiction, Gene Editing Is Now a Looming Reality". In that year, Chinese scientist He Jiankui claimed to have altered the DNA of two embryos using rGE with CRISPR/Cas9. These embryos developed into twins, Lulu and Nana, who were born in October 2018 with a genome modified to be resistant to HIV. Ultimately, the most distant horizon, and still hypothetical, in the development of ARTs is the possibility of a complete extrauterine pregnancy, namely, complete ectogenesis, which would allow unprecedented control over the embryo and fetus throughout gestation.

These and other reproductive technologies have the potential to radically transform our understanding of parenthood and our relationship with progeny. Paraphrasing Jürgen Habermas from two decades ago, whose words are now more relevant than ever, the development of ARTs compels future parents to view their offspring not just as the unpredictable result of evolution but also as the potential outcome of their own choices (Habermas, 2003).

Alongside the tendency to view ARTs as tools that extend, and will continue to extend, the procreative freedom of future parents, there is another perspective to consider. Some authors argue that these techniques not only increase freedom to choose over certain procreative aspects previously left to chance, but also highlight new moral obligations in light of the increased control prospective parents would have in the procreative context. Therefore, considering the prospects for the development of ARTs – both the most immediate and plausible and the most remote – it becomes crucial to examine the relationship between freedom and responsibility in procreation. As a matter of fact, through the tools of bioethical–philosophical reflection, this book aims to rethink the concept of procreative responsibility in light of the continuous development of ARTs, investigating the moral obligations of those who are about to procreate. To do this, I will propose a reflection within the person-affecting morality, according to which, roughly speaking, what matters morally is not producing a state of affairs with greater well-being, but the actions and omissions that can affect or at least be directed at actual people. I use this approach because person-affecting reasons meet with particular consensus from different moral perspectives. Moreover, this approach is generally used to emphasize procreative freedoms rather than procreative duties; nonetheless, I will argue that, in light of the technological developments of ARTs, this could be no longer the case.

Although I will consider several ARTs currently available and those that could be available in the future, the primary attention will be paid to rGE; this technique has the potential to be an actual revolution in the field of human reproduction in the near future; furthermore, it also presents morally significant differences from a person-affecting perspective compared to the techniques currently available and mostly used, which will be at the center of the reflection of this book. However, the reflections that I will suggest for rGE also have value for other ARTs that will be discussed within this work. Therefore, these implications will be adequately mentioned. In particular, in Chapter 7, I will devote some discussions to procreative responsibility in light of the future and hypothetical availability of complete ectogenesis.

The general thesis I will present and defend is what I call the Greater Moral Obligation View. Given the peculiarities of some ARTs that could have future clinical applications, particularly rGE, prospective parents will face a greater moral obligation toward their offspring compared to the moral constraints encountered in a context where only current ARTs are available. This will inaugurate a substantial expansion of procreative responsibility, an unprecedented change since the introduction of ARTs decades ago.

Specifically, this book comprises seven chapters and is structured as follows. The first two chapters serve as an introductory function, laying the groundwork for the following normative proposals. In Chapter 1, I will present in detail the ARTs currently available and those that could be available in the future. In this way, I intend to provide the reader with an accessible overview of the current possibilities and limits, as well as what the prospects of such practices might be. Those who already have some understanding of these techniques can skip this part and begin reading the book from Section 1.3 where I explicit the ethical and technical assumptions of this work.

Chapter 2 offers a philosophical analysis of the concept of responsibility and its relationship with technological development, applying this reflection in the procreative context. I will provide an original taxonomy of procreative duties, proposing a morally relevant distinction between parental responsibility, procreative responsibility, procreative-parental responsibility, and reproductive responsibility. Then, I will specify how the procreative responsibility prescriptions should be conceived considering the moral complexity of human reproduction and the controversial definition of disability.

Based on the technical and conceptual considerations proposed in the first two chapters, the remaining chapters constitute the ethical–philosophical core of this work. Here, I will analyze the arguments proposed in the literature to assess whether there is an actual extension of procreative responsibility in light of new technological possibilities at the beginning of life and, from this, provide an original proposal. The main focus will be on moral duties toward offspring, trying to answer the question "what do we owe our future children?". However, I will also devote some attention to other types of procreative prescriptions in order to highlight the need to combine different types of reasons to propose a complete account of procreative responsibility.

In Chapter 3, I will present and reject the Principle of Procreative Beneficence, exploring some of its challenges already discussed in the debate and proposing new ones, arising from the problematic relationship between impersonal reasons and the concept of person-affecting harm in procreative choices assumed by the principle's advocates. I will also devote some attention to the impersonal nature of this principle. To unpack this aspect, I will discuss the Non-Identity Problem and some of the failing strategies trying to solve it, including the controversial perspective of impersonal harm in maximizing and consequentialist terms.

In Chapter 4, I will introduce what I call the consequences-based person-affecting morality, considering it a solid starting point for discussing procreative obligations. In this context, I will propose the Greater Moral Obligation View, stating that the availability of rGE on early embryos brings forth brand new moral obligations compared to techniques such as preimplantation or post-implantation genetic testing. In this regard, I will introduce and discuss two original procreative-parental responsibility models: the Bold Restriction of Procreative Autonomy and the Mild Restriction of Procreative Autonomy. While the first argues that the Greater Moral Obligation View applies to all prospective parents, the second maintains that only those prospective parents who are already within the IVF process encounter new procreative duties. I will argue that, within a consequences-based person-affecting perspective, we have reason to embrace only the Mild Restriction of Procreative Autonomy while dismissing the Bold Restriction of Procreative Autonomy. After applying such reflection on other ARTs that exhibit morally relevant similarities with rGE, I will acknowledge that in order to have a more comprehensive understanding of moral duties implied by procreative responsibility, we should integrate the prescriptions of the Mild Restriction of Procreative Autonomy with others coming from reproductive responsibility, which shifts the focus from duties toward offspring to duties toward third parties.

In Chapter 5, I recognize that the Greater Moral Obligation View relies on the fundamental assumption that rGE is a non-identity-affecting procedure. Then, I will consider and reject several objections to this assumption: the identity objection, the critique of the necessity of rGE for the existence of the modified individual, the "artificially constrained future" objection, and the critique of the inevitability of Preimplantation Genetic Diagnosis.

In Chapter 6, I will claim that the Mild Restriction of Procreative Autonomy has been framed in Chapter 4 as a negative procreative-parental responsibility model since it prescribes only to avoid harmful conditions in the future child. However, since I argue that it is plausible that procreative-parental responsibility can have not only a negative dimension but also a positive one, I investigate whether the Greater Moral Obligation View implies that future parents are also morally obliged to enhance their future child through rGE, analyzing the Child's Right to an Open Future argument.

Finally, in Chapter 7, I will consider not only the consequences of procreative choices, as done in the previous chapters, but also the moral relevance of intentions and attitudes for procreative responsibility, in a way compatible with person-affecting morality. I will introduce the Parent–Child Relationship argument to suggest that prospective parents are committed to having certain parental intentions and attitudes in the procreative context. Therefore, I will argue that, in this context, the Greater Moral Obligation View demands more than what is required by the Mild Restriction of Procreative Autonomy: all prospective parents may have moral reasons to choose reproduction via ARTs, such as rGE and ectogenesis, rather than sexual intercourse. The Bold Restriction of Procreative Autonomy will thus be rehabilitated.

References

Habermas, J. (2003). *The future of human nature* (1st ed.). Polity Press.
Haimov-Kochman, R., Sciaky-Tamir, Y., & Hurwitz, A. (2005). Reproduction concepts and practices in ancient Egypt mirrored by modern medicine. *European Journal of Obstetrics, Gynecology, and Reproductive Biology*, 123(1), 3–8.
Klipstein, S. (2017). Parenting in the age of preimplantation gene editing. *The Hastings Center Report*, 47, S28–S33.

1 Current and Future Assisted Reproductive Technologies and Prenatal Treatments

In this chapter, I aim to describe currently available Artificial Reproductive Technologies (ARTs) and prenatal treatments, as well as those that could be available in the future. Their characteristics are relevant not only from a scientific standpoint but also from a moral perspective. Therefore, understanding their functioning is fundamental to exploring ethical issues related to procreative responsibility. This chapter is structured as follows: in Section 1.1, I will present already available ARTs, such as *In Vitro* Fertilization (IVF) with embryo transfer and Preimplantation Genetic Diagnosis (PGD). Subsequently, I will introduce prenatal genetic testing, genetic carrier testing, and fetal therapy. In addition, I will explore the relatively new Mitochondrial Replacement Therapy (MRT), a pioneering practice available for a few years that shares similarities with one of the practices currently under development, the genetic modification of gametes, embryos, or fetuses through genome editing. Since it represents a primary focus of this book due to its profound implications on procreative responsibility, I will pay particular attention to the modification of early embryos *in vitro* through reproductive Genome Editing (rGE). In addition to genome editing, in Section 1.2, I will present *In Vitro* Gametogenesis (IVG) and ectogenesis, both in its partial and complete form. Finally, following the discussion of the ARTs mentioned above, in Section 1.3, I will clarify the technical and ethical assumptions of this work. To this end, I will endorse the Pragmatic Optimism approach, systematically introduced in the literature by Nicholas Agar (2004), highlighting its utility in addressing ethical issues related to procreative responsibility in future contexts.

1.1 Currently Available Techniques

1.1.1 *In Vitro Fertilization with Embryo Transfer*

IVF is a technique that involves the artificial fertilization of an oocyte, followed by the transfer of the resulting embryo into the uterus. This

DOI: 10.4324/9781032654683-2

process first involves monitoring and stimulating ovulation, subsequently removing one or more oocytes from the uterus and placing them in a Petri dish to allow sperm to penetrate the oocyte. After the zygote formation, it is allowed to develop in culture for 2–6 days before being transferred into the uterus, hoping that it will implant into the uterine wall and that pregnancy will effectively begin.

IVF is called homologous when the male and female gametes belong to the unborn child's parents. In contrast, it is called heterologous when the genetic material from at least one individual outside the couple intending to have the child is utilized. IVF is mainly used for infertility treatment.[1] It is, in fact, an effective tool in cases where a person with a uterus has problems with the fallopian tubes, making *in vivo* fertilization difficult. IVF is also helpful in addressing male infertility, where the quality of the sperm is poor or the number of sperm is reduced. In these cases, IVF occurs through Intracytoplasmic Sperm Injection (ICSI), which entails inserting individual sperm into the ooplasm of the oocytes. Through a testicular biopsy, ICSI allows the selection of the best quality sperm, which will be used to fertilize the oocytes. Moreover, if combined with sperm donation or egg donation, IVF allows people with a uterus who have already reached menopause or have a partner affected by sterility to become pregnant.

The first *in vitro* baby, Louise Brown, was born in July 1978 in England, thanks to the technique developed by scientists Patrick Steptoe and Robert Edwards; for developing this technique, Edwards was awarded the Nobel Prize for Medicine in 2010.[2] IVF had a relatively low success rate in the first years after Louise Brown's birth (Edwards et al., 1980). However, this technique has been significantly improved thanks to technological development and scientific advancements in recent years. According to a recent report from the Human Fertilisation and Embryology Authority (HFEA) (2020), in the United Kingdom, the success rate of IVF for patients using their gametes has significantly increased over the last 20 years for all females under 43 years. Moreover, the success rate has tripled for females under 35 years. In general, the birth rate per transferred embryo remains modest: in 2018, only 23% of transferred embryos developed until birth.[3]

To address the initial low success rates, the transfer of multiple embryos was introduced, necessitating ovarian stimulation, even aggressive, to produce more oocytes.[4] This brought to light two main complications: multiple pregnancies and ovarian hyperstimulation syndrome (Niederberger et al., 2018).

Multiple pregnancies are correlated with an increased risk of pregnancy termination, obstetric complications, prematurity, and neonatal morbidity, with possible long-term damage to the unborn child. For this reason, usually, no more than three fertilized embryos are simultaneously introduced into the uterus to ensure a certain probability of pregnancy and, at the same time, avoid the excessive risk of multiple pregnancies. Another promising strategy to prevent multiple pregnancies is to transfer a single embryo into the uterus after assessing its quality, usually through a morphological evaluation, i.e., a procedure performed through a microscope to evaluate, among other factors, the symmetry of the embryo, the presence of more than one nucleus in the blastomeres that make up the embryos, and the presence of free extracellular cytoplasmic material devoid of nuclei (fragmentation) (Machtinger & Racowsky, 2013). In light of recent technological developments in embryo selection, cryopreservation, and embryonic culture, some have even argued for the need to use single embryo transfer as a standard strategy in IVF (Cutting, 2018; Kissin et al., 2015). Single embryo transfer is now a common practice in Europe. Preliminary findings from the European IVF-monitoring Consortium of the European Society of Human Reproduction and Embryology (ESHRE) indicate that in 2020, approximately 57.6% of all IVF and ICSI procedures in Europe used the transfer of a single embryo. This is an increase from 2019, when the figure was slightly above 55.4% (Smeenk, 2023). A morally significant aspect in this context is the fate of embryos not transferred into the uterus: surplus embryos could be cryopreserved and used for future pregnancies of the individuals who produced the embryo employing IVF, scientific research purposes, or even donation.[5]

As for the ovarian hyperstimulation syndrome, it is a syndrome that may result from ovarian stimulation, which can, in its most severe forms, cause abdominal pain, nausea, vomiting, and hospitalization. Over the years, the pathophysiology has been better understood, describing its symptoms and applying methods for its management. Fortunately, in the last decade, the risk factors have been almost wholly described, and preventive measures have been successfully employed, thereby avoiding the manifestation of the syndrome in nearly all females who have undergone IVF (Pellicer et al., 2019).

Aside from the complications described above, it is essential to highlight that ovarian stimulation can be a physically burdensome practice, as it implies taking hormonal drugs. This adds to the potential physical stress caused by the invasive procedures involved in oocyte retrieval and the subsequent transfer of embryos into the uterus. The IVF burdens are not only physical but also psychological: undergoing reproduction cycles that are not successful and considering the possibility of not being able to become pregnant can cause anxiety and concerns (Verhaak et al., 2005), which add to the strong stress already caused by the infertility situation that drives the couple or the individual reproducer to undergo IVF (Al-Inany et al., 2006). However, the use of this technique is steadily increasing and is now generally accepted: in 2020, it was estimated that more than 8 million individuals were born using IVF (Lui Yovich, 2020).

1.1.2 *Preimplantation Genetic Diagnosis*

PGD is an auxiliary procedure to IVF that allows the identification of specific genetic characteristics in early embryos obtained *in vitro* before uterine transfer. It is mainly used to select embryos that do not have genetic mutations that could reasonably lead to the onset of genetic diseases during the unborn child's life. However, as we will see, this practice can also have other applications.

The first applications of PGD took place at the end of the 1980s. Initially, this technique was rarely used: from 1990 until 2004, births after PGD were about a thousand (Verlinsky et al., 2004). Subsequently, the numbers have increased significantly and continue to rise. In 2020, according to the 2020 Assisted Reproductive Technology Fertility Clinic Success Rates Report (2022), PGD was used in 48% of IVF cycles in the United States that transferred at least one embryo.

The diagnosis generally involves the biopsy of early embryos to obtain the genetic material to be analyzed. PGD can be performed using various technologies, such as fluorescent *in situ* hybridization, polymerase chain reaction, and, the more recent and advanced technique, next-generation sequencing.

PGD could theoretically be performed at all stages of embryo development before implantation. However, three approaches are generally used. The most classic form is the embryo biopsy on the third day after sperm penetrates the oocyte. In this case, the procedure is performed on embryos composed of eight cells, removing one, involving minimal risks related to the possible future development of the embryo. The second method is the polar body biopsy, where the genetic material is taken from the polar bodies, namely, cells that develop during oogenesis but are not reproductively functional because they cannot be fertilized. Although this approach is much less invasive, it yields less reliable results. Finally, to overcome some problems related to the small amount of tissue analyzable in the first method, it has been proposed to perform the biopsy on the embryo at the blastocyst stage, that is, five or six days after fertilization, where the cells that compose it are about two hundred. Although this method is not free from technical problems related to the very advanced stage at which the test is performed, it provides reliable results and, according to some experts, it may become the most used technique to perform PGD (Thornhill, 2018). However, to date, the most widely used approach remains biopsy on the embryo on the third day after fertilization. Current PGD procedures allow for error rates (resulting in misdiagnosis) as low as 1–3% (Carvalho et al., 2020). Therefore, PGD is highly reliable; although this tool was not considered a viable substitute for prenatal screening in the past, according to some authors, this technique now represents a real alternative (Albujja et al., 2023).

Although commonly known as PGD, the International Glossary of In-fertility and Fertility proposed a new term to encompass preimplantation genetic screening for aneuploidy (Zegers-Hochschild et al., 2017). Indeed, the term "screening" is inappropriate in defining this procedure since, gen-erally, it indicates the identification of at-risk individuals in a given group who might benefit from a test. However, genetic tests performed before implantation require invasive intervention, and therefore, using the word "screening" can be misleading (Simpson et al., 2019). Consequently, it was decided to use the term Preimplantation Genetic Testing (PGT). In this work, however, I use PGD and PGT interchangeably.

Presenting the new nomenclature allows for a better understanding of the specific functions of different types of preimplantation tests. Indeed, we can distinguish at least three different procedures that fall within the definition of PGT: (a) PGT-A is a procedure that identifies aneuploid embryos – i.e., embryos that present a variation in the "normal" number of chromosomes, that is, the diploid set $2n = 46$ – and thus select euploid embryos for transfer, improving pregnancy rates. Euploid embryos have a higher likelihood of implanting and developing into a complication-free pregnancy; (b) PGT-M is a procedure that identifies monogenic diseases in the embryo that are caused by mutations in a single gene; this technique is used for testing certain cancer predisposition genes, such as BRCA1 and BRCA2 for breast and ovarian cancer. In recent years, there has been a growing discourse on the use of PGT-M for conditions with lower pen-etrance (Kuliev & Rechitsky, 2017; Lemke & Rüppel, 2019); finally, (c) PGT-Sr is a procedure that identifies any structural chromosome anomaly, such as translocations, inversions, duplications, insertions, and deletions (Zegers-Hochschild et al., 2017).

Therefore, PGD has a broad spectrum of clinical applications, ranging from the study of genetic diseases to the study of chromosomal imbalances. However, this technique can also be used for other purposes. For instance, PGD enables the selection of the future child's sex. In this regard, it is worth remembering that the first PGD usage, which took place in 1989 in London at Hammersmith Hospital, was precisely a sex selection for medi-cal reasons. Researcher Elena Kontogianni managed to identify the sex in embryos derived from five couples at risk of X-linked recessive hereditary diseases like color blindness, Duchenne muscular dystrophy, hemophilia A, and ichthyosis. X-linked hereditary diseases originate from mutations on the X sex chromosome. Similar to other genetic conditions, X-linked diseases can be transmitted from parents to offspring, adhering to either dominant or recessive inheritance patterns. If the traits tied to the dis-ease are dominant, the pathologies will be present in both sexes. However, the manifestation differs when the traits are recessive. Males, with their XY sex chromosomes, are more commonly affected by recessive X-linked disorders due to the absence of a second X chromosome, which might carry a healthy allele to mask the effect of a mutated gene. Conversely, females, with their XX chromosomes, often become carriers without displaying symptoms, as a normal allele on their second X chromosome can commonly mask the mutated gene. Thus, by identifying and transferring only female embryos in the uterus, the likelihood of X-linked recessive hereditary diseases in offspring is significantly reduced.

Thus, sex selection can be helpful to avoid transferring embryos with certain pathologies into the uterus; however, this practice can also be performed for non-medical reasons, namely, to fulfill the couple's or single reproducer's desire to have a child of a particular sex. Sex selection for non-medical reasons has animated ethical and legal debate in past years, and in many countries, such as Italy, the United Kingdom, and Germany, the practice is still illegal. In contrast, the procedure is legal in the United States, where demand for it is steadily increasing. Evidence for this trend is the increase in supply or the number of clinics that offer PGD and sex selection for non-medical reasons: while the percentage was 42% in 2006 (Baruch et al., 2008), it rose to 72.2% in 2017 (Capelouto et al., 2018).

The same research that revealed the number of clinics for sex selection in 2006 also highlighted another important use of PGD, which is more controversial and will be extensively discussed in this book, namely, to resort to PGD to seek not to avoid selecting embryos with some genetic disease but to actively search for traits *generally* considered disabilities, such as deafness and achondroplasia. In 2006, 3% of fertility clinics in the United States had provided such service to couples intending to select an embryo with a disability (Baruch et al., 2008). I have not found other studies that track these data in subsequent years; however, this evidence is sufficient to argue that this phenomenon exists and that there are reasons to discuss it from an ethical standpoint.

A further application of PGD – that is not directly aimed at selecting an embryo free from genetic diseases or chromosomal alterations and also at the center of bioethical debate – aims to select and transfer into the uterus one or more embryos that are immunocompatible with a relative who needs genetic material (Robinson & Inquiry, 2002; Sheldon & Wilkinson, 2004; Spriggs & Savulescu, 2002; Taylor-Sands, 2015). Even though it is not widespread, this application, as in the case of selecting for disability, is not merely a theoretical case: in 2000, Jack and Lisa Nash, an American couple, gave birth to a son, Adam, who was selected through PGD to be compatible with his sister Molly for a bone marrow donation. Molly was unfortunately afflicted with Fanconi anemia, a disease that causes genomic instability. Clinical characteristics of Fanconi anemia include bone marrow failure and a high predisposition to cancer.

In the future, PGD could provide information not only about genetic diseases but also about polygenic traits, such as intelligence, and behavioral or aesthetic characteristics; consequently, this additional information could be used to make procreative choices. Indeed, in recent years, there has been increasing discussion, also in public debate (Pagnaer et al., 2021), about PGT for polygenic disorders, often referred to as PGT-P, which involves embryo profiling for various complex diseases and attributes, including intelligence (Treff, Eccles, et al., 2019; Treff, Zimmerman, et al., 2019). This approach has already been brought to market by Genomic Prediction Inc., a US-based company, offering couples the option to assess the polygenic risk of embryos for complex traits such as intellectual disability (Lemieux, 2019). Although the relationship between genetic basis and behavioral traits is not yet clear, and it is known that most phenotypic traits depend crucially on a series of environmental factors, studies suggest that some phenotypic behavioral characteristics, such as the propensity to practice extreme sports (Thomson et al., 2013) or having a higher level of intelligence (Sniekers et al., 2017), may have a genetic basis. However, even assuming that knowledge in the field of genetics provides more information about some behavioral traits, it is at least doubtful that PGD can be an effective tool since this procedure seems to have limited utility in selecting polygenic traits (Karavani et al., 2019). In other words, selecting the "tallest" or "most intelligent" embryo might be of little use since its characteristics would only be slightly superior to those of the other embryos produced.

1.1.3   *Prenatal Testing*

In addition to IVF and PGD, there is a set of techniques aimed at monitoring and detecting genetic, physiological, and anatomical problems during the development of the fetus in the mother's womb. These techniques cannot be strictly classified as ARTs if this term refers to techniques that allow assisted procreation. Nonetheless, prenatal testing can have a decisive impact on procreation, as it provides couples or single reproducers with crucial information that may influence their reproductive choices. Thus, I decided to include prenatal testing in this discussion, as well as other non-strictly assisted reproductive techniques that will be addressed later. In this way, I am giving ARTs a broader definition.

For easily intuitable reasons, prenatal testing is more widespread and widely used than the ones mentioned above. Moreover, the scientific community strongly recommends some diagnostic tests for future mothers. The American College of Obstetricians and Gynecologists guidelines, for example, suggest that all pregnant persons, regardless of age, be offered tests to obtain a definitive diagnosis of certain birth defects of the child (2017).

There are essentially three reasons to perform prenatal testing: (a) to allow timely medical or surgical treatment before or after birth; (b) to give parents the option to interrupt the pregnancy of a fetus with the detected condition, where such possibility is provided by law; and (c) to ensure that parents have the opportunity to prepare psychologically, socially, financially, and medically for a child with health problems or disabilities, or the eventuality of fetal death.

Prenatal testing can be distinguished into two categories: prenatal screening and prenatal diagnosis. A screening test informs prospective parents of the risk of a baby having a certain condition. A diagnostic test, which tends to be more invasive, provides a definitive confirmation or exclusion of a specific condition or disease in the baby.

A widespread invasive diagnostic technique is the karyotype analysis from amniotic fluid, which is retrieved through amniocentesis. This procedure allows transabdominal withdrawal of amniotic fluid from the uterine cavity. Through this procedure, the presence of not only chromosomal diseases at the fetal level but also genetic diseases such as thalassemia, spina bifida, albinism, and muscular dystrophy can be assessed. It can be recommended when there is a suspicion of a genetic or chromosomal condition in the fetus, based on family medical history, maternal age, or abnormal results from other screening tests. The risk of abortion linked to the invasiveness of the technique is calculated at around 0.5% (Salomon et al., 2019). Another prenatal diagnostic technique is chorionic villus sampling, which involves extracting fetal cells from the chorionic villi that constitute the embryonic part of the placenta. Chorionic villus sampling is performed earlier in pregnancy than amniocentesis and can extract more significant amounts of tissue. However, it is more invasive, and the risk of abortion is calculated at around 2–3% (Salomon et al., 2019).

Commonly non-invasive prenatal screening used during pregnancy nowadays includes the examination of the uterus through ultrasound and, in combination, the analysis of biochemical markers in maternal blood. This technique allows for the prediction of the probability of fetal aneuploidies, especially in expectant mothers within age groups associated with lower risks of fetal chromosomal pathologies, who would not usually be candidates for invasive pregnancy monitoring. In this context, it is worth mentioning the possibility of testing fetal DNA through a non-invasive practice called Non-Invasive Prenatal Testing (NIPT). From the first trimester of pregnancy, free fetal DNA in the maternal bloodstream can be retrieved non-invasively and used to study certain fetal pathologies. NIPT, introduced in 2010, has been defined as a "revolutionary" tool (Thomas et al., 2021), as it is extremely sensitive to aneuploidies and, therefore, much more reliable than other non-invasive tests for detecting chromosomal disorders like Down syndrome (Palomaki et al., 2011). NIPT is widely adopted in Europe, Australia, and the United States, although only a few countries have a national policy regulating its use (Gadsbøll et al., 2020). This technique certainly presents several advantages, such as avoiding the risk of unintended pregnancy terminations or reducing the need for invasive practices.

Nonetheless, as with techniques described in previous sections, prenatal testing, especially in non-invasive forms, brings up ethical issues. These are mainly associated with the phenomenon of "normalization" of prenatal tests or the inclination to view prenatal testing as a routine examination (Thomas et al., 2021). Although the discussion of normalization is beyond the scope of this work, it is noteworthy that this issue can also arise with other forms of genetic testing that are conducted even before prospective parents plan to conceive, specifically carrier genetic testing.

1.1.4 Carrier Genetic Testing

Carrier genetic testing is a type of genetic test performed on a potential parent, not on embryos or fetuses. It is used to determine whether an individual is a carrier of a specific gene mutation for certain genetic disorders concerning the so-called reproductive risk, namely, the chance that a reproducer or a couple will have to conceive a child with a genetic disorder. It is mainly used to detect autosomal recessive diseases or X-linked hereditary diseases. This procedure involves a simple blood draw and allows the identification of couples who run the risk of conceiving a child affected by a genetic disease in every pregnancy, even if the partners do not present symptoms of the condition. When both partners are heterozygous for the same autosomal recessive disease, or when the female carries an X-linked hereditary disease, there is a 25% probability of transmitting the disease to the offspring (Wienke et al., 2014). Therefore, carrier genetic testing offers future parents more reproductive options: at-risk couples might choose to resort to IVF and subsequently to PGD to select unaffected embryos; they might conceive using donor gametes; they might conceive naturally and subsequently undergo prenatal diagnosis; they might take the risk and, if necessary, accept the future child's condition; and they might ultimately decide to abstain from reproducing (Chokoshvili et al., 2016). These choices will be at the heart of the reflection of this work and will be analyzed from an ethical point of view in the following chapters.

Carrier genetic testing for some recessive diseases has been available for over 50 years. Already in 1969, testing was available for Tay–Sachs disease, a lethal childhood neurodegenerative disease particularly prevalent in the Ashkenazi Jewish population (Kaback, 2000). Subsequently, carrier testing was also used to detect other recessive disorders, including fragile X syndrome, spinal muscular atrophy, and cystic fibrosis. Although today the test is usually offered to future parents considered to be at higher risk, generally based on the presence of individuals affected by the diseases mentioned above in their ancestry or ethnicity, recent developments in the field of genetics have made it possible to detect hundreds of recessive disorders through a single test, the so-called universal carrier test. Some commercial companies have already begun to provide this type of test, and it is reasonable to expect that in the coming years, the use of the universal carrier test will increase (McGowan et al., 2013).

1.1.5 Fetal Therapy

Fetal therapy refers to a set of interventions performed to treat congenital diseases in the fetus while it is still *in utero*. The purpose of fetal therapy may be to achieve a complete prenatal cure, alleviate severe pediatric developmental or functional deficiencies, or optimize the fetal transition to extrauterine life. In the same way as prenatal testing, this procedure cannot be defined as an ART in the narrowest sense. However, it is one of the most relevant practices for the ethical discussion that I will propose in the following chapters.

Various fetal therapy interventions can be categorized based on their invasiveness. The least invasive procedure involves using a needle guided by ultrasound to perform, for instance, an intrauterine transfusion or collect a fetal blood sample. Fetal procedures also include fetoscopic procedures through which small incisions are made to resolve, for example, issues related to umbilical cord occlusion. The most invasive fetal therapy is open fetal surgery, which involves fully opening the uterus to operate on the fetus to remove, for example, a teratoma, a tumor of the embryonic tissues (Moon-Grady et al., 2017).

Although historically the main aim of fetal therapy was to treat conditions that could compromise the life of the fetus, since the 2000s therapeutic interventions for non-lethal conditions have also been accepted (Cortes & Farmer, 2004). To date, fetal therapy is particularly effective and used to treat twin-to-twin transfusion syndrome in a minimally invasive way, a rare condition that can occur in monochorionic pregnancies. In this situation, where two or more twins share the same placenta and the same chorion, there is an alteration of fetal circulation, which leads to an unequal distribution of the amount of blood that goes from the placenta to the twins (Codsi & Audibert, 2019). In addition, fetal therapy is now employed to address conditions like spina bifida, which aids in lowering the chances of hydrocephalus and enhancing motor functions in affected children (Adzick, 2013), and congenital diaphragmatic hernia, presenting an opportunity to enhance pulmonary outcomes for infants with severe manifestations (Deprest & Flake, 2022).

Fetal therapy is not without risks: first, in some of its forms, it is a highly invasive intervention and potentially harmful to the pregnant person. Moreover, a significant issue currently remains: even in cases of fetoscopy, the relatively high risk of preterm rupture of membranes often leads to premature births. Fetal therapy is, therefore, a very complex and delicate practice, especially considering that the invasive interventions mentioned do not involve just one patient but two: the fetus and the mother. The fetal interventions considered standard today are very few, and many applications are still experimental; these consistently aim to make fetal therapy as minimally invasive as possible. Thus, the risks and benefits of the practices in question must be constantly weighed to promote the health of the mother and fetus.

Fetal therapy, however, has promising prospects, which depend not only on technological developments but also on advancements in related fields of knowledge, such as neonatology and regenerative medicine. The actual future of fetal surgery likely resides in stem cells and gene therapy, which might not only improve the outcomes of fetal therapy for structural anomalies but also broaden the spectrum of possible applications to genetic disorders (Shear & Massa, 2021; Sparks, 2021).

1.1.6 Mitochondrial Replacement Therapy

The most recent ART available today is MRT. Through this technique, it is possible to prevent the transmission of mitochondrial diseases from mother to child, such as Leigh and Pearson syndrome. Mitochondrial diseases are primarily hereditary neuromuscular diseases caused by alterations in the functioning of mitochondria, cellular organelles present in eukaryotic organisms, which are commonly considered the "powerhouse" of the cell as they produce the energy needed for vital cellular functions (Tachibana et al., 2009). Mitochondrial DNA is different from the nuclear DNA of cells and is almost entirely inherited from the mother. MRT, therefore, aims to prevent the transmission of mitochondrial DNA and can occur in two different ways: pronuclear transfer and maternal spindle transfer.

Pronuclear transfer requires the creation of two zygotes through IVF, one with the gametes of the couple intending to have a child and the other with a donated egg and the father's sperm. In this scenario, the first zygote has defective mitochondria since it was created with the mother's oocyte, while the second zygote has healthy mitochondria having been created with a donated oocyte. On the first day after fertilization, the maternal and paternal pronuclei are removed from both zygotes. The enucleated zygote produced with the mother's oocyte and the pronuclei of the cell produced with the donor's oocyte are discarded. Subsequently, the pronuclei of the couple intending to have a child are transferred to the enucleated cell produced with the donor's oocyte and the male partner's sperm. The reconstructed zygote, which possesses healthy mitochondria, can then be transferred to the mother's uterus or a surrogate (Craven, Elson, et al., 2011; Craven, Tuppen, et al., 2010).

The maternal spindle transfer technique initially involves obtaining two oocytes: one from the patient carrying a mitochondrial disease, who intends to have a child, and the other from a healthy donor. Using a micromanipulation system and polarized light microscopy, the mitotic spindle of the carrier patient's oocyte is isolated and then extracted. Subsequently, the extracted genetic material is transferred to the donor's oocyte, from which the nucleus was previously extracted. The resulting oocyte is then fertilized with sperm, creating the embryo, which, before transfer to the uterus, undergoes PGD to check for mitochondrial mutations (Board on Health Sciences Policy et al., 2016). MRT thus produces an individual genetically related to three people: the biological father and mother, and a mitochondrial DNA donor, even though the mitochondrial DNA of the donor will constitute only about 0.15% of the child's DNA.

MRT is particularly useful in cases where a carrier person with a uterus wants to conceive a child who does not have a mitochondrial disease. Although PGD is still an option in these cases, the diagnostic technique does not always guarantee that the future individual will not be affected by a mitochondrial disease. According to Joanna Poulton and colleagues, when mutations are new or uncommon, there is not enough clinical data available to effectively guide the couple's decision through PGD (Poulton et al., 2009). For the same reason and because the PGD process is used in mitochondrial therapy, it is worth noting that this technique cannot currently guarantee the prevention of transmitting mitochondrial diseases but can only reduce the risk significantly. Furthermore, due to the possibility of genetically correlating the future individual with two different females, MRT would allow homosexual female couples to have a child genetically related to both (Cavaliere & Palacios-González, 2018).

This technique is not free from risks. In addition to those already mentioned for IVF and PGD, there are other factors to consider. First, zygote and oocyte manipulations could have adverse effects on the resulting embryo: there would indeed be a risk that the oocytes might mature abnormally or that fertilization could occur irregularly. Second, since the mitochondria in the final oocyte will come from a third party, different from the two parties whose DNA is in the nucleus, and since nuclear DNA encodes some genes that produce some of the proteins used by the mitochondria, there might be a risk of "mito-nuclear" interactions. Lastly, MRT does not completely eliminate the mitochondrial DNA from the disease carrier in the future individual, although the remaining amount is less than 2% (Human Fertilisation and Embryology Authority, 2016).

After a thorough analysis, the HFEA has determined that the aforementioned mitochondrial therapy techniques used in UK clinics are sufficiently advanced to manage associated risks. As a result, in 2016, the HFEA decided to make the procedure available in the United Kingdom, specifically for couples for whom PGD is unlikely to be effective in producing a child free from the mother's mitochondrial disease (2016). In 2023, the HFEA announced that at least one child had been born in the United Kingdom using MRT (Callaway, 2023), even though the first baby conceived using this method was born to a Jordanian family receiving treatment from a US-based team in Mexico back in 2016. To date, MRT is not widespread, because it is extremely expensive and meets a rather meager demand (Rulli, 2017). The United Kingdom and Australia – starting in March 2022 – are the only countries to have regulated MRT, although it has been used, as already mentioned, in Mexico and also Greece and Ukraine (Sharma et al., 2020).

1.2   Technologies Potentially Available in the Future

1.2.1   In Vitro Gametogenesis

The first technique I present that may be available in the future for clinical application is IVG, which aims to create *in vitro* gametes from non-sexual cells. According to several authors, such technology could change the paradigm of genetic parenthood (I. G. Cohen et al., 2017; Notini et al., 2020).

We can distinguish at least two IVG techniques: the first strategy involves the creation of induced Pluripotent Stem Cells (iPSCs), namely, genetically reprogramming a somatic cell from one of the parent-would-be to become iPSCs, and differentiating these iPSCs into gametes and then, following the routine IVF procedures, combining them with the complementary gametes of the partner (Hendriks et al., 2015). This results in a child who shares 50% of the genetic heritage with one partner and 50% with the other; the second strategy requires the creation of an embryo via somatic cell nuclear transfer. Such a technique consists of taking a denucleated oocyte and implanting a donor nucleus from a somatic cell, resulting in a cloned embryo with the parents' DNA, except 0.15% of mitochondrial DNA. Persons with a uterus could use their own oocytes for this procedure so that there would be no "foreign" mitochondria present in the resulting child. After the blastocyst stage, the developing germ cells would then be harvested from the embryo's inner cell mass and cultured to maturity. Once the mature gametes are formed, they can be combined with the partner gametes (Hendriks et al., 2015).

Research on mice has shown promising results: several methods have produced functional gametes in rodent models (Hayashi, Ogushi, et al., 2012; Hayashi, Ohta, et al., 2011; Nagamatsu & Hayashi, 2017).

Concerning humans, Japanese scientists have managed to generate human oogonia from iPSCs, germ cells that are fundamental to oogenesis as they differentiate into primary oocytes that begin the meiotic process (Yamashiro et al., 2018). While challenges persist in human studies, evidence indicates that, with further refinement, it might be possible to derive functional human eggs and sperm from iPSCs in the foreseeable future (I. G. Cohen et al., 2017; Kushnir et al., 2022).

IVG may have different advantages in the reproductive context. First, it could be used to overcome infertility or even sterility problems of opposite-sex couples, in which one or both partners are affected by these conditions, to have genetically related children. Accordingly, it facilitates postmenopausal motherhood, allowing people to reproduce later. Another potential clinical application of IVG is enabling same-sex couples to have a child who is equally genetically related to both partners, and even multiplex parenting, namely, groups of more than two individuals procreate together. Moreover, the techniques employed in IVG also allow "solo" genetic parenthood (solo IVG) in cases in which both gametes are created stemming from a single individual. Finally, and quite relevant for this work, IVG could also be used to create a significant number of embryos, expanding and accelerating the genetic selection of offspring with desired characteristics (Suter, 2016).

1.2.2 Genome Modification: From Gene Therapy to Genome Editing

Another procedure that could potentially revolutionize our understanding of reproduction in the future is undoubtedly the modification of the human genome on gametes, embryos, or fetuses. The idea of replacing a non-functioning part of DNA with a healthy part was introduced by Theodore Friedmann and Richard Roblin (Friedmann & Roblin, 1972). Friedman and Roblin's arguments were based on the significant scientific progress of the 1970s regarding the study of DNA and, in particular, on the discovery of "restriction endonucleases", enzymes capable of cutting DNA at specific sites. Another crucial discovery was recombinant DNA: Paul Berg, in 1972, isolated a gene capable of developing tumors in mice and chemically welded it to a virus that infects bacteria. Thus, such viral DNA could integrate entirely or partially with the mice's DNA. Recombinant DNA is therefore based on relatively simple criteria: (a) identifying a gene, (b) cutting and isolating it from the DNA molecule, (c) joining the substitute gene to a vector, and (d) transferring it inside a receiving cell (Refolo et al., 2017). Thanks to these studies, there has been significant progress in molecular biology and genetic engineering methods that have allowed cloning, gene sequencing, and, above all, the development of a therapeutic practice called gene therapy.

Gene therapy entails the introduction of genetic material, which has been previously incorporated into appropriate vectors, including viruses or plasmids, into target patient cells. In this way, the normal functions of an individual affected by a genetic disease caused by the malfunctioning or absence of a specific gene are restored. The first case of gene therapy in humans, although only partially successful, was carried out in 1990 by William French Anderson (McCain, 2005): he treated a girl affected by severe combined immunodeficiency (SCID), a deficiency of the enzyme adenosine deaminase that compromises the immune system. However, in its early years, gene therapy suffered from various technical problems, compromising its actual success. For instance, the vector inserted inside the cells could damage a part of "good" DNA: this occurred in France during attempts at SCID therapy. On that occasion, the patients undergoing the treatment contracted leukemia due to a mutation of specific genes of the white blood cells (Hacein-Bey-Abina et al., 2008). Over the years, new methods have been developed that can reduce this kind of problem, thus increasing the precision of the therapy. In this context, we can introduce a new declination of gene therapy called genome editing.

Genome editing involves inserting, deleting, modifying, or replacing DNA sequences within an organism's genome. Although genome modification has been possible since the development of gene therapy, there are some differences between traditional gene therapy and genome editing. First, traditional gene therapy techniques do not offer any control over where DNA modification occurs within the genome. The viral vector cannot insert the code fragment precisely but in more or less random sites. Gene therapy, therefore, has higher risk elements compared to genome editing. Second, standard gene therapy only allows adding DNA segments to the genome, for example, inserting an extra copy of a gene. Genome editing, instead, enables researchers to delete and replace specific parts with other sequences, considerably expanding possible interventions. To date, the most advanced and used genome editing technique is CRISPR/Cas (Doudna, 2020): the CRISPR/Cas system is a tool that allows DNA modification in living cells with high precision. The two components of the system, CRISPR and Cas, are part of an adaptive immune system found in nature in bacteria and archaea. The acronym "CRISPR" stands for "clustered regularly interspaced short palindromic repeats" and refers to specific parts of bacterial DNA sequence discovered for the first time in 1987. The name "Cas" stands for "CRISPR-associated" and refers to a class of bacterial proteins that include nucleases, i.e., proteins that can perform the cutting of the DNA double helix.

The CRISPR/Cas system distinguishes itself from other genome editing methods due to its ease of use. Especially when using the Cas9 protein as a nuclease, the CRISPR system provides researchers with a simple method for creating organisms with an altered genome (Ran et al., 2013). Thanks to this method, it is possible to replace a gene in the DNA sequence of a target cell with another inserted into the cell. CRISPR/Cas9 is not the only method used for genome editing. There are other techniques, such as ZFNs and TALENs; however, they are less user-friendly compared to CRISPR/Cas9. These methods require the development of specific targeting proteins for each new application of the technique, a much more laborious and error-prone phase compared to the RNA-based approach offered by the CRISPR/Cas9 system (Doudna, 2020). The limited cost of CRISPR/Cas9 and its ease of use have allowed its wide application in basic research and its extensive spread (Baltimore et al., 2015).

Notwithstanding, CRISPR/Cas9 still has significant problems; from various experiments, it has been noted that the DNA cutting is not always precise and can sometimes bring off-target changes in sites where it was not intended to modify the DNA; in other words, CRISPR could lead to unintentional interventions, for example, a change in the gene B expression when the target was changing gene A expression (Guttinger, 2017). Off-target changes could, however, be reasonably solved by scientific and technological developments in the field of biotechnologies; the CRISPR/Cas system is indeed continuously improving (Hu & Li, 2022). Furthermore, there is an additional problem given by our lack of knowledge about the human genome: even if the genomic modification were successful, it could predispose the modified individual and their offspring to other genetic conditions (Guttinger, 2017). In general, it is complex to determine if a seemingly successful genome editing treatment could, in the future, cause unforeseen problems at a certain period of the individual's life or that of their progeny. To reduce such problems, scientists should deepen their knowledge about the roles that existing elements of DNA have within the genome and be able to provide a prediction of the behavior of modified DNA sequences.

1.2.2.1 *Somatic and Germline Genome Editing*

There are two types of genome editing: one performed on somatic cells and one performed on germline cells. Both procedures are relevant for this work, although more space will be devoted to presenting germline genome editing.

Somatic genome editing is currently the most studied and experimented with method. It aims to modify the DNA of somatic cells, which make up an organism's body or soma. Somatic cell clusters form the various tissues that, in complex organisms, make up organs and, in turn, systems. In November 2023, the UK's Medicines and Healthcare Products Regulatory

Agency approved using somatic genome editing to treat sickle cell disease and beta-thalassemia (2023).

Germline Genome Editing aims to modify genes present in cells such as sperm and eggs or cells of early embryonic stages. These cells are initially undifferentiated, and only later, during embryonic development, they will differentiate to become specialized somatic cells. Germline modification is transmitted to offspring, unlike somatic cell modification. Advancements in CRISPR technology suggest that, in the foreseeable future, individuals or couples may opt for IVF procedures, subsequently altering the genome of gametes or early-stage embryos before their transfer into the uterus. In light of this, I refer to the utilization of germline genome editing in human reproduction as rGE. For the purpose of this work, my focus will primarily be on rGE in early embryos, as opposed to gametes. In a nutshell, through rGE, we will be able to choose some genetic traits of the future individual directly by modifying *in vitro* human embryos' DNA before transferring them to the uterus.

In the short term, rGE will be particularly effective in treating monogenic genetic diseases, such as Duchenne muscular dystrophy, cystic fibrosis, and Huntington's disease in early embryos (Doudna, 2020; Tang et al., 2017). Note that rGE could be a more effective tool than PGD alone in cases, despite quite rare, where the chances of selecting an embryo unaffected by a mutation for genetic diseases are quite low or null. For example, if one of the future parents is homozygous for a dominant genetic disease, like Huntington's disease, the risk of transmission to offspring is 100% (J. Cohen, 2020); therefore, it would not be possible to obtain an embryo that is not a carrier of the genetic disease through IVF. If both partners in a couple are heterozygous for a dominant genetic disease, the risk of transmission goes up to 75%, so the chances of finding embryos without mutation are low. Another case where PGD is insufficient is when both future parents are homozygous for a recessive genetic disease, meaning both carry two variants of the gene that causes the disease. In these cases, rGE can modify an affected embryo and give birth to a genetically related child free of genetic diseases. Moreover, in a more distant future, it might be possible to prevent polygenic diseases in offspring, that is, diseases that do not depend on a single gene but on the joint effect of various genes, such as hypertension, coronary disease, and diabetes (Savulescu et al., 2015).

As already mentioned in the introduction of this book, the possibility of modifying the genome in early embryos is, in some ways, already a reality: while the first experiments on tripronuclear human embryos only took place in 2015 (Liang et al., 2015), in 2018, Chinese scientist He Jiankui declared that he had modified the genome of twin girls, who were born in October of the same year, with a DNA resistant to HIV (Marchione, 2018). This experiment was strongly condemned by much of the scientific community due to violations of research protocols and the risks of this technique that are still poorly understood. In this regard, it is important to mention that the absence of a functional CCR5 – the gene modified by Jiankui to make the twins HIV–resistant – can increase the risks related to West Nile virus and other viruses (Glass et al., 2006; Greely, 2019). In light of this, some scientists have proposed a moratorium (Lander et al., 2019) to temporarily ban rGE applications.

In general, rGE encounters technical hurdles that will have to be solved before its application at a clinical level. In addition to the problems related to off-target cuts, there is another quite complex problem to consider: for rGE to be widely effective, certain diseases or genetic characteristics in an embryo could be known before making modifications. This would require a preimplantation diagnostic tool like PGD, capable of detecting any genetic diseases or specific genetic traits in the embryo before operating with genome modification. rGE, at least in its early applications, should be performed at a stage prior to the first cell division or immediately afterward to avoid mosaicism issues, i.e., the presence, in a multicellular organism, of two or more different genetic lines. However, although it is theoretically possible to perform PGD at any stage of embryonic development, with the current state of the art, performing genetic tests on embryos at this stage would mean destroying the embryo. Moreover, especially when not all embryos are likely carriers of a genetic disease, it does not even seem desirable to perform genome editing blindly and then perform PGD later; this would risk damaging embryos without genetic mutations unless rGE reaches levels of effectiveness and safety that avoid this scenario. In light of this, the first available clinical applications will be those in which there is reasonable certainty that all embryos produced in IVF have a certain genetic characteristic that is desired to be modified. However, it is desirable that future scientific developments in genome editing techniques and PGD resolve these difficulties to expand the application spectrum of rGE (Hershlag & Bristow, 2018).

As previously said, rGE is not the only type of genetic editing relevant to procreative responsibility. Although the applications of somatic genome editing mostly take place in already developed people, we can imagine that in the future, it will be possible to act on the individual's somatic cells in the prenatal phase to effectively solve genetic diseases that may affect the fetus' development. Clearly, editing the fetus' genome is a more invasive practice compared to rGE on early embryos, as it should take place *in vivo*, i.e., in the mother's uterus; moreover, the problem of mosaicism, we already discussed for rGE, remains also for this application of Somatic Genome Editing.

Finally, from an even more distant perspective, but in principle not unfeasible, both types of genetic modification discussed here could have applications not so much aimed at curing genetic diseases, but at modifying some aesthetic traits or enhancing complex traits, such as intelligence, height, and memory, in embryos that have the potential to develop into a person who already possesses the characteristics that fall within the normal functioning of the human species.

1.2.3 The Artificial Uterus and Ectogenesis

A further technology that could have disruptive effects on human reproduction in the future is the artificial uterus, a device that allows the development of an embryo outside a female organism, which would normally carry the pregnancy to term. The role of the artificial uterus should be to provide nourishment and oxygen to the fetus and dispose of waste material. It should also provide immune protection against diseases by transmitting antibodies to the embryo or fetus, as occurs when the fetus is in the maternal womb. The introduction of the artificial uterus can have two significant consequences: premature babies before the 22nd week could increase their chances of survival, which are currently almost null; moreover, this technique might enable an entire pregnancy to begin and end without the embryo being implanted in the maternal uterus. In other words, the artificial uterus would allow what John Burdon Sanderson Haldane defined in 1924 as ectogenesis, which can be categorized as partial ectogenesis if referring to the first application mentioned, or complete ectogenesis if referring to the second application.

Concerning partial ectogenesis, current techniques could allow clinical use of the artificial uterus in this sense within a decade. A 2017 study reports a lamb fetus's development and birth after being inserted into an extrauterine support system for four weeks (Partridge et al., 2017). In this context, researchers at the Children's Hospital of Philadelphia designed and used a sort of plastic bag, the so-called biobag, capable of mimicking the protection offered by the maternal placenta. The biobag was filled with an electrolytic solution that mimics the amniotic fluid, in which the fetus, taken from the maternal womb equivalent to the 23rd week of human gestation, was inserted. A tube was then connected to the developing fetus to simulate the functions of the umbilical cord. This allowed the blood to be filtered from waste and carbon dioxide, enriching it with nutrients and oxygen. In 2023, scientists at the Children's Hospital of Philadelphia sought permission from the US Food and Drug Administration to initiate the first human clinical trials for a device they had developed, termed the Extra-uterine Environment for Newborn Development, or EXTEND (Kozlov, 2023).[6] Also, a perinatal life support aimed at helping human fetuses to survive even before the 22nd week of life is under development through a Horizon project coordinated by the Eindhoven University of Technology.[7]

Regarding complete ectogenesis, actual clinical applications are certainly more distant and hypothetical compared to partial ectogenesis. There are technical problems related to the complexity of the natural uterus and the biological relationship between mother and fetus. For instance, there are significant issues in the hormonal stability of the fetus and the use of artificial nutrition, which would not allow for the survival of the fetus or the newborn. In addition, there are issues concerning the oxygenation of the embryo, for which the technique of extracorporeal membrane oxygenation has been proposed. This functioning technique has successfully kept goat fetuses alive for up to 237 hours in the amniotic tank (Sakata et al., 1998). However, using such practice in the weeks preceding the 32nd exposes a high risk of intraventricular hemorrhage.

Even though in 2016 two studies were published concerning the development of embryos for 12–13 days within an ecto-uterine environment, problems persist related to the development of embryos that are a few days old (Deglincerti et al., 2016; Shahbazi et al., 2016). Nonetheless, such experiments would have significant consequences on legislation currently in force in 12 countries, which states that allowing the development of an embryo for more than 14 days without implanting it in the uterus or destroying it is forbidden. Encouraging signals come from animal experimentation: recently, researchers from the Weizmann Institute of Science have effectively developed mouse embryos up to late organogenesis or until the stage of forming hind limbs (Aguilera-Castrejon et al., 2021).

The potential advantage of ectogenesis is to allow the fetus to develop in an environment not influenced by possible maternal diseases, alcohol, or drugs that the pregnant person might use. Moreover, there would be no risks of an immune reaction against the embryo or fetus that might otherwise result from insufficient gestational immune tolerance. This practice could also more easily allow surgical or manipulative interventions on embryos aimed at resolving the future individual's genetic defects, without these interventions being invasive for the mother. Lastly, ectogenesis would also have the advantage of avoiding physical burdens on the pregnant person, albeit at the cost of foregoing an essential aspect of motherhood itself, namely, the symbiotic relationship between the mother and fetus before the latter's birth.

1.3 Ethical and Technical Assumptions: Pragmatic Optimism

After having discussed current and future ARTs and prenatal treatment, it is vital to illustrate two categories of assumptions without which this work would have no reason to exist.

First, an ethical assumption must be made. Even before raising issues related to procreative responsibility, the aforementioned techniques may raise ethical problems regarding their own permissibility and the consequences of their implementation.

Concerning IVF and PGD, for instance, some argue that these techniques are ethically problematic as they involve the disposal of embryos that are not transferred *in utero* or their use for experimentation. This argument is based on the belief that the embryo should be always treated, from its conception, as a person; therefore, discarding an embryo due to its genetic heritage or using it for experimentation would be a direct assault on human dignity. There are also people who tolerate homologous IVF but are against some heterologous IVF because, among other applications, they would allow homosexual couples to have a child genetically related to at least one of them. This argument assumes, quite controversially, that it is morally wrong for a homosexual couple to have children. MRT and especially the potential future use of IVG might prompt similar worries, as they could challenge the traditional ideas of parenthood by enabling same-sex couples, multiple parents, and single individuals to procreate (Baylis, 2018; Notini et al., 2020; Palacios-González & Cavaliere, 2019; Segers et al., 2019).

Moreover, others might argue that in some applications of ARTs, there is a devaluation of women and sometimes outright exploitation of the female body. This argument is supported by the ethics of sexual difference, aimed at particularly valuing the public role, as well as the private one, of peculiar experiences related to procreation: pregnancy, breastfeeding, care for the young, and relationships. This approach critiques patriarchal society and science (Holmes & Purdy, 1992). In this line, there is the risk that overly invasive reproductive techniques cause excessive objectification and exploitation of women's bodies. Accordingly, society must prevent new technologies from strengthening the exclusively reproductive role that patriarchy reserves for them. Supporters of this thesis criticize, for example, egg donation, which relegates the woman to a merely reproductive function; altruistic surrogacy, which treats the woman as a mere fetal container; and even more commercial surrogacy, which would constitute a real and precise exploitation of reproductive labor: it would be alienated labor since the fruits of such labor are enjoyed by others. Women would devalue their role, while the child would be treated like a commodity. Ectogenesis is also criticized in this line, which would once again ignore the peculiarity of female reproductive work, as is sex selection through PGD, since it would discriminate against women and strengthen the values of patriarchy.[8]

Despite these arguments primarily focusing on the category of women, it is essential to recognize that they may also apply, at least partially, to individuals who do not define themselves as women but who have the biological capacity for pregnancy. To ensure inclusivity, throughout this book, I will primarily use terms like "pregnant person" or "pregnant individuals" instead of "pregnant woman". This language choice is in line with respecting the identities and experiences of all individuals capable of pregnancy, including those who are transgender, non-binary, or gender non-conforming, while still critically engaging with the ethical considerations surrounding ARTs.

Regarding the possibility of rGE, various ethical issues have been raised in the debate.[9] First, its usage would be controversial since it would not be possible to obtain the consent of the future individual (Collins, 2015). Another criticism assumes that rGE vexes nature: allowing the manipulation of life itself, rGE would redesign the natural world and threaten its integrity. Here, the central element is that altering DNA is morally ambiguous. Indeed, the concept of nature is often associated with the moral judgment of "good," but such an attitude proves to be inappropriate (Holtug, 1997). This argument can also be understood in other terms: it would be morally problematic to manipulate human nature because it is impossible to predict such an act's potentially catastrophic consequences.[10]

Moreover, even assuming the acceptability of genome editing to prevent the onset of some genetic diseases in the future individual, according to some, it would still be mainly problematic because it would trigger a slippery slope toward morally contentious applications (Walton, 2017). Allowing rGE for ends that we might roughly define here as "therapeutic" would necessarily lead to the legitimacy of using such a technique for enhancing purposes, thereby inaugurating new eugenics.[11] Other authors might not necessarily be committed to supporting the slippery slope argument as presented but still claim that rGE to enhance future offspring is morally problematic because it conflicts with the self-understanding of future individuals as members of the human species (Habermas, 2003), it is against human dignity (Kass, 2004), it may undermine appreciation of the gifted character of human talents and achievements (Sandel, 2009), or it would lead to a class division in a society where the previous generation would in some ways be obsolete compared to the next because of the continuous development of genetic enhancement technologies (Sparrow, 2019).

Finally, there could be problems with access to the aforementioned reproductive technologies (Tonkens, 2018): the high cost could limit their use only to the wealthiest. In this context, it is essential to ask whether there is a right to reproduction and biological parenthood, understood as an individual right to perpetuate one's genes, and whether this right should be understood by State authority as a negative right or even as a positive right (I. G. Cohen & Jackson, 2020; Hall, 2022). Furthermore, some techniques may be consistent with the right to a decent minimum level of healthcare, and this may pose an allocative justice problem (Buchanan et al., 2000). On the contrary, some might argue that techniques such as

IVF, PGD, MRT, or rGE cannot be considered strictly akin to therapy and instead represent new ways of reproducing in continuity with the medicine of desires (Rulli, 2017, 2019).[12]

The ethical problems mentioned are just some of those raised by new technological possibilities at the beginning of life. This work does not aim to respond to these objections and thus justify the moral legitimacy of ARTs presented in the previous sections. Therefore, I limit myself to assuming that the currently available ARTs and those that will be available in the future should be considered tools available to reproducers and ethically acceptable concerning the issues mentioned in this section.

Moreover, in what follows, the human embryo will not be considered an entity with full moral status nor a depository of intrinsic consideration. However, this does not imply that some considerations that will be proposed cannot be embraced and shared even by those who argue that the embryo should always be considered as if it were a person and, therefore, a repository of human dignity. To avoid issues related to reproductive justice, I assume that the various present and future techniques are accessible to the entire population, cheap, and legal.

However, more than such assumptions is required. Although I assumed that practices must be considered legal, accessible, and economically and ethically legitimate, it is worth emphasizing that they must also be safe and sufficiently effective. As some data reported in previous sections show, the presented techniques are often poorly effective, and risks to the pregnant person are certainly not excluded. Furthermore, practices such as rGE are still quite far from clinical application, and some authors even argue that the development of such technologies is not even very useful and desirable (Rulli, 2019). Furthermore, concerning genetic enhancement, there is no certainty that technological development and knowledge of the human genome can lead to effectively modifying genes and thus achieving a significant phenotypic change in the intelligence or character of the future individual. In the same line, the development prospects for ectogenesis are mostly speculative.

In light of this uncertainty, one might wonder why we should now reflect on the ethical issues of remote future scenarios or even merely possible ones. To answer this question, I believe it can be helpful to introduce the conceptual tool of Pragmatic Optimism, according to which it is better to have principles to face situations that prove impossible than not having principles for situations in which we suddenly find ourselves (Agar, 2004). From this perspective, we should provide ourselves with "moral insurance". To do so, we must think beyond the limits of current scientific knowledge and technological possibilities. What we need are principles for situations that may never occur but whose possibility cannot be excluded given our current state of knowledge. Therefore, to investigate issues related to future procreative responsibility, we should embrace some optimism about the greater accuracy and efficacy of the currently available reproductive techniques and the future possibility of genome editing (both on the somatic line and the germline) applied to human reproduction and of ectogenesis, as well as genetic enhancement. In this context, the ethical considerations related to procreative responsibility must be understood "in principle" since they are dependent on technologies and their "in principle" possibilities. Pragmatic Optimism intentionally abstracts from risk considerations and feasibility to focus on the objectives that motivate the development of these technologies (Agar, 2004). It allows the kind of moral discussion we must have *before* technologies are adopted or reach sufficient levels of efficacy.

Although Pragmatic Optimism encourages a broad view of scientific possibilities, it is not an approach capable of predicting bizarre and implausible developments of reproductive technologies. In line with Agar, proposals that transcend the scientific or metaphysical limits of the techniques should be excluded from moral consideration (Agar, 2004). From this perspective, we should not embrace a form of extreme genetic determinism, according to which all phenotypic traits would depend only on the individual's genetic heritage. For example, some complex phenotypic characteristics cannot be explained solely on the basis of the genome but also depend on interaction with the environment. However, it is also true that some genetic variants provide certainty or significant predisposition for some phenotypic traits.

In summary, adopting Pragmatic Optimism means presenting the technologically ideal scenario to assess the expansion of procreative responsibility in light of the development of the techniques as mentioned earlier. In this scenario, IVF has reached quite high success rates – equal, if not superior, to gestation *in utero* – and it is possible to perform PGD effectively and safely at any stage of embryonic development. Through the latter and developments in genomic knowledge, it is possible to identify most human genes and their functions effectively. In other words, it is possible to identify genes for monogenic and polygenic diseases and identify genes related to complex phenotypic traits such as intelligence. Thanks to the development of genome editing and fetal therapy, it is possible to modify early embryos or fetuses not only to avoid genetic diseases but also to enhance some human characteristics without such changes having unwanted side effects during the life of the future individual. Regarding rGE, the problems related to mosaicism have been solved, and finally, ectogenesis guarantees both the partial and the complete development of pregnancy outside the maternal uterus, allowing greater control over the health of the future individual.

This scenario does not claim to be a prediction. However, in light of the technological developments described above, it seems plausible to argue that at least part of it can reasonably be realized. Considering technologically ideal scenarios can thus prepare us for the many possible futures that technologies involved in the reproduction process might create.

Notes

1 Infertility refers to the situation in which a heterosexual couple is unable to achieve pregnancy after a year of unprotected intercourse. It can generally be resolved and is related to one or more interfering factors. Infertility is different from sterility, which is a permanent, non-resolvable physical condition of the male or female (or both) that makes conception impossible.
2 Steptoe was unable to collect the award with Edwards as he passed away in 1988.
3 Despite other HFEA reports on fertility treatments have been published, I mainly refer to the 2018 data, since outcomes from 2019 to 2021 have not yet been validated due to the COVID-19 pandemic and large-scale work to upgrade the HFEA data submission system and migrate data to a new database. As HFEA reports, this means that some data in this report are preliminary and cannot be compared to other reports, see HFEA (2023).
4 In the early years of IVF, eggs were retrieved without first proceeding with this procedure.
5 As will be highlighted in Section 1.3, in this work I will not discuss these issues. In this regard, see, among others, Grobstein (1982).
6 The FDA discussed the case at the end of September. At the time of writing, a decision has not been reached.
7 https://perinatallifesupport.eu
8 For a more recent contribution on feminist perspective and ARTs, see Lie and Lykke (2019).
9 For a general discussion of the ethical problems of the rGE, see, among others, Gyngell et al. (2017).
10 I tried to reply to these arguments in Battisti (2019a).
11 I presented and attempted to answer this argument in Battisti (2019b). For further discussion on the "new eugenics argument" and ARTs, see Camporesi (2015).
12 For a discussion, see Cavaliere (2018).

References

Adzick, N. S. (2013). Fetal surgery for spina bifida: Past, present, future. *Seminars in Pediatric Surgery, 22*(1), 10–17.
Agar, N. (2004). *Liberal eugenics: In defence of human enhancement.* John Wiley & Sons.
Aguilera-Castrejon, A., Oldak, B., Shani, T., Ghanem, N., Itzkovich, C., Slomovich, S., Tarazi, S., Bayerl, J., Chugaeva, V., Ayyash, M., Ashouokhi, S., Sheban, D., Livnat, N., Lasman, L., Viukov, S., Zerbib, M., Addadi, Y., Rais, Y., Cheng, S., ... Hanna, J. H. (2021). Ex utero mouse embryogenesis from pre-gastrulation to late organogenesis. *Nature.* https://doi.org/10.1038/s41586-021-03416-3
Al-Inany, H. G., Abou-Setta, A. M., & Aboulghar, M. (2006). Gonadotrophin-releasing hormone antagonists for assisted conception. *Cochrane Database of Systematic Reviews, 3*, CD001750.

Albujja, M. H., Al-Ghedan, M., Dakshnamoorthy, L., & Pla Victori, J. (2023). Preimplantation genetic testing for embryos predisposed to hereditary cancer: Possibilities and challenges. *Cancer Pathogenesis and Therapy*. https://doi.org/10.1016/j.cpt.2023.05.002

American College of Obstetricians and Gynecologists. (2017). Committee opinion no. 690 summary: Carrier screening in the age of genomic medicine. *Obstetrics and Gynecology, 129*(3), 595–596.

Baltimore, D., Berg, P., Botchan, M., Carroll, D., Charo, R. A., Church, G., Corn, J. E., Daley, G. Q., Doudna, J. A., Fenner, M., Greely, H. T., Jinek, M., Martin, G. S., Penhoet, E., Puck, J., Sternberg, S. H., Weissman, J. S., & Yamamoto, K. R. (2015). Biotechnology. A prudent path forward for genomic engineering and germline gene modification. *Science (New York, NY), 348*(6230), 36–38.

Baruch, S., Kaufman, D., & Hudson, K. L. (2008). Genetic testing of embryos: Practices and perspectives of US in vitro fertilization clinics. *Fertility and Sterility, 89*(5), 1053–1058.

Battisti, D. (2019a). Il genome editing con CRISPR/Cas9: Implicazioni tecniche ed etiche. *Etica per Le Professioni, 3*, 105–113.

Battisti, D. (2019b). Genome editing: Slipping down toward Eugenics? *Medicina Historica, 3*(3), 206–218.

Baylis, F. (2018). 'No' to lesbian motherhood using human nuclear genome transfer. *Journal of Medical Ethics, 44*(12), 865–867.

Buchanan, A., Brock, D. W., Daniels, N., & Wikler, D. (2000). *From chance to choice*. Cambridge University Press.

Callaway, E. (2023). First UK children born using three-person IVF: What scientists want to know. *Nature, 617*(7961), 443–444.

Camporesi, S. (2015). "Stop this talk of new eugenics!"-reframing the discourse around reproductive genetic technologies to choose disabilities as practices of ethical self-formation. *Western Humanities Review, 69*(3), 135–147.

Capelouto, S. M., Archer, S. R., Morris, J. R., Kawwass, J. F., & Hipp, H. S. (2018). Sex selection for non-medical indications: A survey of current pre-implantation genetic screening practices among U.S. ART clinics. *Journal of Assisted Reproduction and Genetics, 35*(3), 409–416.

Carvalho, F., Coonen, E., Goossens, V., Kokkali, G., Rubio, C., Meijer-Hoogeveen, M., Moutou, C., Vermeulen, N., De Rycke, M., & ESHRE PGT Consortium Steering Committee. (2020). ESHRE PGT Consortium good practice recommendations for the organisation of PGT. *Human Reproduction Open, 2020*(3). https://doi.org/10.1093/hropen/hoaa021

Cavaliere, G. (2018). Genome editing and assisted reproduction: Curing embryos, society or prospective parents? *Medicine, Health Care, and Philosophy, 21*(2), 215–225.

Cavaliere, G., & Palacios-González, C. (2018). Lesbian motherhood and mitochondrial replacement techniques: Reproductive freedom and genetic kinship. *Journal of Medical Ethics, 44*(12), 835–842.

Centers for Disease Control and Prevention, American Society for Reproductive Medicine, Society for Assisted Reproductive Technology. (2022). *2020 Assisted reproductive technology fertility clinic success rates report*. https://www.cdc.gov/art/reports/2020/pdf/Report-ART-Fertility-Clinic-National-Summary-H.pdf

Chokoshvili, D., Janssens, S., Vears, D., & Borry, P. (2016). Designing expanded carrier screening panels: Results of a qualitative study with European geneticists. *Personalized Medicine, 13*(6), 553–562.

Codsi, E., & Audibert, F. (2019). Fetal surgery: Past, present, and future perspectives. *Journal d'obstetrique et Gynecologie Du Canada* [Journal of Obstetrics and Gynaecology Canada], 41(Suppl 2), S287–S289.

Cohen, I. G., Daley, G. Q., & Adashi, E. Y. (2017). Disruptive reproductive technologies. *Science Translational Medicine, 9*(372). https://doi.org/10.1126/scitranslmed.aag2959

Cohen, I. G., & Jackson, E. (2020). Introduction to the right to procreate and assisted reproductive technologies. In Hervey T. K., Orentlicher D., *The Oxford Handbook of Comparative Health Law* (pp. 988-C47.P17). Oxford University Press.

Cohen, J. (2020). Narrow path charted for editing genes of human embryos. *Science (New York, NY), 369*(6509), 1283.

Collins, F. S. (2015). *Statement of NIH Funding of Research Using Gene-Editing Technologies in Human Embryos.* https://www.nih.gov/about-nih/who-we-are/nih-director/statements/statement-nih-funding-research-using-gene-editing-technologies-human-embryos.

Cortes, R. A., & Farmer, D. L. (2004). Recent advances in fetal surgery. *Seminars in Perinatology, 28*(3), 199–211.

Craven, L., Elson, J. L., Irving, L., Tuppen, H. A., Lister, L. M., Greggains, G. D., Byerley, S., Murdoch, A. P., Herbert, M., & Turnbull, D. (2011). Mitochondrial DNA disease: New options for prevention. *Human Molecular Genetics, 20*(R2), R168–R174.

Craven, L., Tuppen, H. A., Greggains, G. D., Harbottle, S. J., Murphy, J. L., Cree, L. M., Murdoch, A. P., Chinnery, P. F., Taylor, R. W., Lightowlers, R. N., Herbert, M., & Turnbull, D. M. (2010). Pronuclear transfer in human embryos to prevent transmission of mitochondrial DNA disease. *Nature, 465*(7294), 82–85.

Cutting, R. (2018). Single embryo transfer for all. *Best Practice & Research. Clinical Obstetrics & Gynaecology, 53*, 30–37.

Deglincerti, A., Croft, G. F., Pietila, L. N., Zernicka-Goetz, M., Siggia, E. D., & Brivanlou, A. H. (2016). Self-organization of the in vitro attached human embryo. *Nature, 533*(7602), 251–254.

Deprest, J., & Flake, A. (2022). How should fetal surgery for congenital diaphragmatic hernia be implemented in the post-TOTAL trial era: A discussion. *Prenatal Diagnosis, 42*(3), 301–309.

Doudna, J. A. (2020). The promise and challenge of therapeutic genome editing. *Nature, 578*(7794), 229–236.

Edwards, R. G., Steptoe, P. C., & Purdy, J. M. (1980). Establishing full-term human pregnancies using cleaving embryos grown in vitro. *BJOG: An International Journal of Obstetrics and Gynaecology, 87*(9), 737–756.

Friedmann, T., & Roblin, R. (1972). Gene therapy for human genetic disease? *Science (New York, NY), 175*(4025), 949–955.

Gadsbøll, K., Petersen, O. B., Gatinois, V., Strange, H., Jacobsson, B., Wapner, R., Vermeesch, J. R., NIPT-map Study Group, & Vogel, I. (2020). Current use of noninvasive prenatal testing in Europe, Australia and the USA: A graphical presentation. *Acta Obstetricia et Gynecologica Scandinavica, 99*(6), 722–730.

Glass, W. G., McDermott, D. H., Lim, J. K., Lekhong, S., Yu, S. F., Frank, W. A., Pape, J., Cheshier, R. C., & Murphy, P. M. (2006). CCR5 deficiency increases risk of symptomatic West Nile virus infection. *The Journal of Experimental Medicine, 203*(1), 35–40.

Greely, H. T. (2019). CRISPR'd babies: Human germline genome editing in the 'He Jiankui affair.' *Journal of Law and the Biosciences, 6*(1), 111–183.

Grobstein, C. (1982). The moral uses of "spare" embryos. *The Hastings Center Report, 12*(3), 5–6.

Guttinger, S. (2017). Trust in science: CRISPR–Cas9 and the ban on human germline editing. *Science and Engineering Ethics.* https://doi.org/10.1007/s11948-017-9931-1

Gyngell, C., Douglas, T., & Savulescu, J. (2017). The ethics of germline Gene Editing. *Journal of Applied Philosophy, 34*(4), 498–513.

Habermas, J. (2003). *The future of human nature* (1st ed.). Polity Press.

Hacein-Bey-Abina, S., Garrigue, A., Wang, G. P., Soulier, J., Lim, A., Morillon, E., Clappier, E., Caccavelli, L., Delabesse, E., Beldjord, K., Asnafi, V., MacIntyre, E., Dal Cortivo, L., Radford, I., Brousse, N., Sigaux, F., Moshous, D., Hauer, J., Borkhardt, A., … Cavazzana-Calvo, M. (2008). Insertional oncogenesis in 4 patients after retrovirus-mediated gene therapy of SCID-X1. *The Journal of Clinical Investigation, 118*(9), 3132–3142.

Hall, G. A. (2022). Reproduction misconceived: Why there is no right to reproduce and the implications for ART access. *Journal of Medical Ethics.* https://10.1136/jme-2022-108512.

Hayashi, K., Ogushi, S., Kurimoto, K., Shimamoto, S., Ohta, H., & Saitou, M. (2012). Offspring from oocytes derived from in vitro primordial germ cell-like cells in mice. *Science (New York, NY), 338*(6109), 971–975.

Hayashi, K., Ohta, H., Kurimoto, K., Aramaki, S., & Saitou, M. (2011). Reconstitution of the mouse germ cell specification pathway in culture by pluripotent stem cells. *Cell, 146*(4), 519–532.

Hendriks, S., Dancet, E. A. F., van Pelt, A. M. M., Hamer, G., & Repping, S. (2015). Artificial gametes: A systematic review of biological progress towards clinical application. *Human Reproduction Update, 21*(3), 285–296.

Hershlag, A., & Bristow, S. L. (2018). Editing the human genome: Where ART and science intersect. *Journal of Assisted Reproduction and Genetics, 35*(8), 1367–1370.

Holmes, H. B., & Purdy, L. M. (Eds.). (1992). *Feminist perspectives in medical ethics.* Indiana University Press.

Holtug, N. (1997). Altering humans—the case for and against human gene therapy. *Cambridge Quarterly of Healthcare Ethics: CQ: The International Journal of Healthcare Ethics Committees, 6*(2), 157–174.

Hu, Y., & Li, W. (2022). Development and application of CRISPR-Cas based tools. *Frontiers in Cell and Developmental Biology, 10.* https://doi.org/10.3389/fcell.2022.834646

Human Fertilisation and Embryology Authority. (2016). *Scientific review of the safety and efficacy of methods to avoid mitochondrial disease through assisted conception.* https://www.hfea.gov.uk/media/2611/fourth_scientific_review_mitochondria_2016.pdf

Human Fertilisation and Embryology Authority. (2020). *Fertility treatment 2018: Trends and figures.* https://www.hfea.gov.uk/about-us/publications/research-and-data/fertility-treatment-2018-trends-and-figures/

Human Fertilisation and Embryology Authority. (2023). *Fertility treatment 2021: Preliminary trends and figures.*

Kaback, M. M. (2000). Population-based genetic screening for reproductive counseling: The Tay-Sachs disease model. *European Journal of Pediatrics, 159*(Suppl 3), S192–S195.

Karavani, E., Zuk, O., Zeevi, D., Barzilai, N., Stefanis, N. C., Hatzimanolis, A., Smyrnis, N., Avramopoulos, D., Kruglyak, L., Atzmon, G., Lam, M., Lencz, T., & Carmi, S. (2019). Screening human embryos for polygenic traits has limited utility. *Cell, 179*(6), 1424–1435.e8.

Kass, L. R. (2004). *Life liberty & the defense of dignity.* Encounter Books.

Kissin, D. M., Boulet, S. L., & Adashi, E. Y. (2015). Yes, elective single-embryo transfer should be the standard of care. In Carrell, D. T., Schlegel, P. N., Racowsky C., Gianaroli L., (Eds.), *Biennial Review of Infertility Volume 4* (pp. 177–187). Springer International Publishing.

Kozlov, M. (2023). Human trials of artificial wombs could start soon. Here's what you need to know. *Nature, 621*(7979), 458–460.

Kuliev, A., & Rechitsky, S. (2017). Preimplantation genetic testing: Current challenges and future prospects. *Expert Review of Molecular Diagnostics, 17*(12), 1071–1088.

Kushnir, V. A., Smith, G. D., & Adashi, E. Y. (2022). The future of IVF: The new normal in human reproduction. *Reproductive Sciences (Thousand Oaks, CA), 29*(3), 849–856.

Lander, E. S., Baylis, F., Zhang, F., Charpentier, E., Berg, P., Bourgain, C., Friedrich, B., Joung, J. K., Li, J., Liu, D., Naldini, L., Nie, J.-B., Qiu, R., Schoene-Seifert, B., Shao, F., Terry, S., Wei, W., & Winnacker, E.-L. (2019). Adopt a moratorium on heritable genome editing. *Nature, 567*(7747), 165–168.

Lemieux, J. (2019). The risky business of embryo selection: Genomic prediction adds polygenic risk scores to the preimplantation genetic screening menu. *Genetic Engineering and Biotechnology News, 39*(4), 20–22.

Lemke, T., & Rüppel, J. (2019). Social dimensions of preimplantation genetic diagnosis: A literature review. *New Genetics and Society, 38*(1), 80–112.

Liang, P., Xu, Y., Zhang, X., Ding, C., Huang, R., Zhang, Z., Lv, J., Xie, X., Chen, Y., Li, Y., Sun, Y., Bai, Y., Songyang, Z., Ma, W., Zhou, C., & Huang, J. (2015). CRISPR/Cas9-mediated gene editing in human tripronuclear zygotes. *Protein & Cell, 6*(5), 363–372.

Lie, M., & Lykke, N. (2019). *Assisted reproduction across borders feminist perspectives on normalizations, disruptions and transmissions.* Routledge.

Lui Yovich, J. (2020). Founding pioneers of IVF update: Innovative researchers generating livebirths by 1982. *Reproductive Biology, 20*(1), 111–113.

Machtinger, R., & Racowsky, C. (2013). Morphological systems of human embryo assessment and clinical evidence. *Reproductive Biomedicine Online, 26*(3), 210–221.

Marchione, M. (2018, November 26). *Chinese researcher claims first gene-edited babies.* Associated Press. https://www.apnews.com/4997bb7aa36c45449b488e19ac83e86d

McCain, J. (2005). The future of gene therapy. *Biotechnology Healthcare*, 2(3), 52.

McGowan, M. L., Cho, D., & Sharp, R. R. (2013). The changing landscape of carrier screening: Expanding technology and options? *Health Matrix (Cleveland, Ohio)*, 23(1), 15–33.

Medicines and Healthcare products Regulatory Agency. (2023). *MHRA authorises world-first gene therapy that aims to cure sickle-cell disease and transfusion-dependent β-thalassemia*. GOV.UK. https://www.gov.uk/government/news/mhra-authorises-world-first-gene-therapy-that-aims-to-cure-sickle-cell-disease-and-transfusion-dependent-thalassemia

Moon-Grady, A. J., Baschat, A., Cass, D., Choolani, M., Copel, J. A., Cromble-holme, T. M., Deprest, J., Emery, S. P., Evans, M. I., Luks, F. I., Norton, M. E., Ryan, G., Tsao, K., Welch, R., & Harrison, M. (2017). Fetal treatment 2017: The evolution of fetal therapy centers – A joint opinion from the international fetal medicine and surgical society (IFMSS) and the north American fetal therapy network (NAFTNet). *Fetal Diagnosis and Therapy*, 42(4), 241–248.

Nagamatsu, G., & Hayashi, K. (2017). Stem cells, in vitro gametogenesis and male fertility. *Reproduction*, 154(6), F79–F91.

Niederberger, C., Pellicer, A., Cohen, J., Gardner, D. K., Palermo, G. D., O'Neill, C. L., Chow, S., Rosenwaks, Z., Cobo, A., Swain, J. E., Schoolcraft, W. B., Fry-dman, R., Bishop, L. A., Aharon, D., Gordon, C., New, E., Decherney, A., Tan, S. L., Paulson, R. J., ... LaBarbera, A. R. (2018). Forty years of IVF. *Fertility and Sterility*, 110(2), 185–324.e5.

Notini, L., Gyngell, C., & Savulescu, J. (2020). Drawing the line on in vitro game-togenesis. *Bioethics*, 34(1), 123–134.

Pagnaer, T., Siermann, M., Borry, P., & Tšuiko, O. (2021). Polygenic risk scoring of human embryos: A qualitative study of media coverage. *BMC Medical Ethics*, 22(1), 125.

Palacios-González, C., & Cavaliere, G. (2019). 'Yes' to mitochondrial replacement techniques and lesbian motherhood: A reply to Françoise Baylis. *Journal of Medical Ethics*, 45(4), 280–281.

Palomaki, G. E., Kloza, E. M., Lambert-Messerlian, G. M., Haddow, J. E., Neveux, L. M., Ehrich, M., van den Boom, D., Bombard, A. T., Deciu, C., Grody, W. W., Nelson, S. F., & Canick, J. A. (2011). DNA sequencing of maternal plasma to detect Down syndrome: An international clinical validation study. *Genetics in Medicine: Official Journal of the American College of Medical Genetics*, 13(11), 913–920.

Partridge, E. A., Davey, M. G., Hornick, M. A., McGovern, P. E., Mejaddam, A. Y., Vrecenak, J. D., Mesas-Burgos, C., Olive, A., Caskey, R. C., Weiland, T. R., Han, J., Schupper, A. J., Connelly, J. T., Dysart, K. C., Rychik, J., Hedrick, H. L., Peranteau, W. H., & Flake, A. W. (2017). An extra-uterine system to physiologically support the extreme premature lamb. *Nature Communications*, 8(1), 15112.

Pellicer, N., Galliano, D., & Pellicer, A. (2019). Ovarian hyperstimulation syndrome. In Leung, P. C. K., & Adashi E. Y., (Eds.), *The ovary* (pp. 345–362). Elsevier.

Poulton, J., Kennedy, S., Oakeshott, P., & Wells, D. (2009). Preventing transmission of maternally inherited mitochondrial DNA diseases. *BMJ*, 338, b94.

Ran, F. A., Hsu, P. D., Wright, J., Agarwala, V., Scott, D. A., & Zhang, F. (2013). Genome engineering using the CRISPR-Cas9 system. *Nature Protocols*, 8(11), 2281–2308.

Refolo, P., Pascali, V. L., & Spagnolo, A. G. (2017). Editing genetico: nuova questione bioetica? [Gene editing: A new issue for Bioethics?]. *Medicina e Morale*, 66(3), 291–304.

Robinson, B. E. S., & Inquiry, P. (2002). Designing a child to save a child. *Philosophical Inquiry*, 24(1), 87–96.

Rulli, T. (2017). The mitochondrial replacement 'therapy' myth. *Bioethics*, 31(5), 368–374.

Rulli, T. (2019). Reproductive CRISPR does not cure disease. *Bioethics*, 33(9), 1072–1082.

Sakata, M., Hisano, K., Okada, M., & Yasufuku, M. (1998). A new artificial placenta with a centrifugal pump: Long-term total extrauterine support of goat fetuses. *The Journal of Thoracic and Cardiovascular Surgery*, 115(5), 1023–1031.

Salomon, L. J., Sotiriadis, A., Wulff, C. B., Odibo, A., & Akolekar, R. (2019). Risk of miscarriage following amniocentesis or chorionic villus sampling: Systematic review of literature and updated meta-analysis. *Ultrasound in Obstetrics & Gynecology: The Official Journal of the International Society of Ultrasound in Obstetrics and Gynecology*, 54(4), 442–451.

Sandel, M. J. (2009). *The case against perfection*. Belknap Press.

Savulescu, J., Pugh, J., Douglas, T., & Gyngell, C. (2015). The moral imperative to continue gene editing research on human embryos. *Protein & Cell*, 6(7), 476–479.

Segers, S., Pennings, G., Dondorp, W., de Wert, G., & Mertes, H. (2019). In vitro gametogenesis and reproductive cloning: Can we allow one while banning the other? *Bioethics*, 33(1), 68–75.

Shahbazi, M. N., Jedrusik, A., Vuoristo, S., Recher, G., Hupalowska, A., Bolton, V., Fogarty, N. M. E., Campbell, A., Devito, L. G., Ilic, D., Khalaf, Y., Niakan, K. K., Fishel, S., & Zernicka-Goetz, M. (2016). Self-organization of the human embryo in the absence of maternal tissues. *Nature Cell Biology*, 18(6), 700–708.

Sharma, H., Singh, D., Mahant, A., Sohal, S. K., Kesavan, A. K., & Samiksha. (2020). Development of mitochondrial replacement therapy: A review. *Heliyon*, 6(9), e04643.

Shear, M. A., & Massa, A. (2021). In utero fetal therapy: Stem cells, cell transplantation, gene therapy, and CRISPR-Cas9. *Clinical Obstetrics and Gynecology*, 64(4), 861–875.

Sheldon, S., & Wilkinson, S. (2004). Should selecting saviour siblings be banned? *Journal of Medical Ethics*, 30(6), 533–537.

Simpson, J. L., Kuliev, A., & Rechitsky, S. (2019). Overview of preimplantation genetic diagnosis (PGD): Historical perspective and future direction. *Methods in Molecular Biology (Clifton, NJ)*, 1885, 23–43.

Smeenk, J. (2023 7). *Assisted Reproductive Technology (ART) in Europe 2020 and development of a strategy of vigilance: Preliminary results generated from European registers by the ESHRE EIM Consortium.* European and Global ART monitoring, Copenhagen. https://www.eshre.eu/ESHRE2023/Media/2023-Press-releases/EIM

Sniekers, S., Stringer, S., Watanabe, K., Jansen, P. R., Coleman, J. R. I., Krapohl, E., Taskesen, E., Hammerschlag, A. R., Okbay, A., Zabaneh, D., Amin, N., Breen,

G., Cesarini, D., Chabris, C. F., Iacono, W. G., Ikram, M. A., Johannesson, M., Koellinger, P., Lee, J. J., ... Posthuma, D. (2017). Erratum: Genome-wide association meta-analysis of 78,308 individuals identifies new loci and genes influencing human intelligence. *Nature Genetics, 49*(10), 1558–1558.

Sparks, T. N. (2021). The current state and future of fetal therapies. *Clinical Obstetrics and Gynecology, 64*(4), 926–932.

Sparrow, R. (2019). Yesterday's child: How gene editing for enhancement will produce obsolescence-and why it matters. *The American Journal of Bioethics: AJOB, 19*(7), 6–15.

Spriggs, M., & Savulescu, J. (2002). Saviour siblings. *Journal of Medical Ethics, 28*(5), 289.

Suter, S. M. (2016). In vitro gametogenesis: Just another way to have a baby? *Journal of Law and the Biosciences, 3*(1), 87–119.

Tachibana, M., Sparman, M., Sritanaudomchai, H., Ma, H., Clepper, L., Woodward, J., Li, Y., Ramsey, C., Kolotushkina, O., & Mitalipov, S. (2009). Mitochondrial gene replacement in primate offspring and embryonic stem cells. *Nature, 461*(7262), 367–372.

Tang, L., Zeng, Y., Du, H., Gong, M., Peng, J., Zhang, B., Lei, M., Zhao, F., Wang, W., Li, X., & Liu, J. (2017). CRISPR/Cas9-mediated gene editing in human zygotes using Cas9 protein. *Molecular Genetics and Genomics: MGG, 292*(3), 525–533.

Taylor-Sands, M. (2015). Summary of saviour siblings. *Journal of Medical Ethics, 41*(12), 926.

Thomas, J., Harraway, J., & Kirchhoffer, D. (2021). Non-invasive prenatal testing: Clinical utility and ethical concerns about recent advances. *The Medical Journal of Australia, 214*(4), 168–170.e1.

Thomson, C. J., Hanna, C. W., Carlson, S. R., & Rupert, J. L. (2013). The -521 C/T variant in the dopamine-4-receptor gene (DRD4) is associated with skiing and snowboarding behavior. *Scandinavian Journal of Medicine & Science in Sports, 23*(2), e108–e113.

Thornhill, A. R. (2018). Genetic analysis of the embryo: Preimplantation genetic diagnosis. In Skinner, M., (Ed.) *Encyclopedia of reproduction* (pp. 215–221). Elsevier.

Tonkens, R. (2018). Infertilitism: Unjustified discrimination of assisted reproduction patients. *Monash Bioethics Review, 35*(1–4), 36–49.

Treff, N. R., Eccles, J., Lello, L., Bechor, E., Hsu, J., Plunkett, K., Zimmerman, R., Rana, B., Samoilenko, A., Hsu, S., & Tellier, L. C. A. M. (2019). Utility and first clinical application of screening embryos for polygenic disease risk reduction. *Frontiers in Endocrinology, 10*, 845.

Treff, N. R., Zimmerman, R., Bechor, E., Hsu, J., Rana, B., Jensen, J., Li, J., Samoilenko, A., Mowrey, W., Van Alstine, J., Leondires, M., Miller, K., Paganetti, E., Lello, L., Avery, S., Hsu, S., & Melchior Tellier, L. C. A. (2019). Validation of concurrent preimplantation genetic testing for polygenic and monogenic disorders, structural rearrangements, and whole and segmental chromosome aneuploidy with a single universal platform. *European Journal of Medical Genetics, 62*(8), 103647.

Verhaak, C. M., Smeenk, J. M. J., van Minnen, A., Kremer, J. A. M., & Kraaimaat, F. W. (2005). A longitudinal, prospective study on emotional adjustment before, during and after consecutive fertility treatment cycles. *Human Reproduction (Oxford, England)*, 20(8), 2253–2260.

Verlinsky, Y., Cohen, J., Munne, S., Gianaroli, L., Simpson, J. L., Ferraretti, A. P., & Kuliev, A. (2004). Over a decade of experience with preimplantation genetic diagnosis: A multicenter report. *Fertility and Sterility*, 82(2), 292–294.

Walton, D. (2017). The slippery slope argument in the ethical debate on genetic engineering of humans. *Science and Engineering Ethics*, 23(6), 1507–1528.

Wienke, S., Brown, K., Farmer, M., & Strange, C. (2014). Expanded carrier screening panels-does bigger mean better? *Journal of Community Genetics*, 5(2), 191–198.

Yamashiro, C., Sasaki, K., Yabuta, Y., Kojima, Y., Nakamura, T., Okamoto, I., Yokobayashi, S., Murase, Y., Ishikura, Y., Shirane, K., Sasaki, H., Yamamoto, T., & Saitou, M. (2018). Generation of human oogonia from induced pluripotent stem cells in vitro. *Science (New York, NY)*, 362(6412), 356–360.

Zegers-Hochschild, F., Adamson, G. D., Dyer, S., Racowsky, C., de Mouzon, J., Sokol, R., Rienzi, L., Sunde, A., Schmidt, L., Cooke, I. D., Simpson, J. L., & van der Poel, S. (2017). The international glossary on infertility and fertility care, 2017. *Human Reproduction (Oxford, England)*, 32(9), 1786–1801.

2 Responsibility, Procreation, and Reproduction

In the previous chapter, I described the currently available Assisted Reproductive Technologies (ARTs) and prenatal treatments and those that might become available in the future. Moreover, I made explicit some technical and ethical assumptions regarding these technologies, which will guide reflections in this work. In this chapter, I will discuss some elements necessary to understanding procreative responsibility, offering a definition of this concept. I will begin by proposing an analysis of the general concept of responsibility (Section 2.1) through a taxonomy that identifies its various uses in ordinary language. While responsibility can be framed both morally and legally, my focus here will be on the moral sense. Moving to Section 2.2, I focus on material capacity, a necessary condition for an agent to be morally responsible for actions, omissions, or states of affairs. Specifically, I will analyze how technological development can lead to an extension of the moral responsibility of agents. I will then apply this argument to the context of human reproduction and the continuous development of ARTs, claiming that some bioethicists argue in favor of what I call "the colonization of reproduction by ethics". With these points in mind, in Section 2.3, I will introduce a definition of the concept of procreative responsibility. This definition is more concerned with creating a formal taxonomy of the potential duties reproducers face in the reproductive context than with investigating and defining its substantial contents, which I will develop in the following chapters of this work. In order to provide this definition, I will also explore how procreative responsibility is related to the less controversial concept of parental responsibility. Therefore, I will distinguish between procreative responsibility and reproductive responsibility, terms generally used interchangeably in the debate. To that aim, I introduce the notions of procreative-parental responsibility, reproductive-parental responsibility, family-based reproductive responsibility, and broad reproductive responsibility. These distinctions allow us to understand the nuances of the various moral duties reproducers might hold in the procreative context. Next, I will explain how to understand such obligation: given the intricate

DOI: 10.4324/9781032654683-3

ethical, social, and psychological aspects of human reproduction, I argue that such procreative duties and obligations should not be viewed as absolutes. Instead, they should carry relative weight and be balanced with other relevant moral reasons at stake. In other words, they should be treated as *prima facie* moral obligations. Finally, in Section 2.4, I will contend that our understanding of procreative responsibility is also shaped by how we define disability, a complex and contentious concept. I will critically analyze both the well-known Medical and Social models of disability, highlighting their significant challenges. Following this, I will present two alternative models that aim to overcome these challenges: the Welfarist and Equal Opportuties models.

2.1   A Taxonomy of the Concept of Responsibility

The term "responsibility" generally refers to a situation in which an agent can be held accountable for their actions or omissions. Having responsibility for an act means being the one who must answer for it (A. Ross, 1992). Evaluating whether a person is responsible for their behavior and holding others or oneself responsible for certain conduct and its consequences is a central aspect not only of academic ethical reflection but also, and above all, of our daily interpersonal relationships. However, the definition of responsibility is far from clear-cut.

It is possible to detect a certain ambiguity in the definition of this concept. In fact, responsibility has been defined as a "slippery" concept due to its multitude of uses (D. Miller, 2001). As Nicole Vincent points out, philosophical discussions often treat responsibility as a uniform and generic concept (Vincent, 2011). On the contrary, there are several ways in which we can refer to the notion of responsibility. For instance, in the debate about free will, we may investigate whether or not the possibility of determinism excludes the moral responsibility of people (Caruso, 2018; Dennett, 2003; Fischer & Ravizza, 1998). This has been one of the predominant ways to address moral responsibility, which has often been seen as a supplementary topic within the free will debate rather than as a distinct field of inquiry (Nelkin & Pereboom, 2022). In the bioethical debate on organ allocation, we may investigate whether the fact that an individual is or is not responsible for their health condition can determine their priority on the waiting list (Donckier et al., 2014; Moss & Siegler, 1991; Senderovich, 2016). Furthermore, this work explores whether advances in reproductive technologies could extend procreative responsibilities. These are just some examples of the different ways in which the concept of responsibility can be understood and investigated in philosophical and bioethical inquiry.

Setting aside the debate about free will and determinism, for the purposes of this work, it is critical to differentiate the various interpretations of responsibility in discussions about moral responsibility. In order to do that, following Vincent, I report the story of Captain Smith:

(1) Smith had always been an exceedingly responsible person, (2) and as captain of the ship he was responsible for the safety of his passengers and crew. But on his last voyage he drank himself into a stupor, (3) and he was responsible for the loss of his ship and many lives. (4) Smith's defense attorney argued that the alcohol and his transient depression were responsible for his misconduct, (5) but the prosecution's medical experts confirmed that he was fully responsible when he started drinking since he was not suffering from depression at that time. (6) Smith should take responsibility for his victims' families' losses, but his employer will probably be held responsible for them as Smith is insolvent and uninsured.[1]

In the story of Captain Smith, Vincent observes up to six different ways of understanding the concept of responsibility (Vincent, 2011). This distinction is a development of the classification already made by Herbert Hart, who only identified four conceptions of responsibility (H. L. A. Hart, 1968/2008). Although the most relevant concepts of responsibility for this work will be those described by Hart, it is helpful – to avoid confusion – to mainly refer to the more complete taxonomy proposed by Vincent, providing some further refinements.

In the first use, the term "responsible" defines Smith's character. As we learn from the story, he was generally considered reliable and able to fulfill his duties. This is what we can refer to as *virtue responsibility*.

The second use of "responsibility" is related to one's role or position. For instance, Smith, as the ship's captain, has obligations to the passengers. *Role responsibility*, also called responsibility-as-moral-obligation (van de Poel, 2011), coincides with obligations and moral principles (Fonnesu, 2018). Sergio Filippo Magni underscores this by stating that such responsibility inherently means having "obligations to someone" (Magni, 2019, p. 80). In this context, the normative aspect of the concept of responsibility is appropriately captured, as the actions or omissions considered are not yet performed or realized; this implies a forward-looking understanding of responsibility. From this perspective, the attribution of role responsibility can provide the agent with reasons for acting or refraining from acting in a certain way. Moreover, role responsibility is a relation between at least two entities (van de Poel, 2011); however, this does not mean that individuals have obligations tied only to the formal role they hold. More specifically, following Ibo van de Poel, saying "A is responsible for X to B" – where A is an agent, X can be actions or states of affairs, and B is the party to whom A has obligations – highlights that we might have distinct responsibilities toward various individuals (van de Poel, 2011). An individual, indeed, can occupy multiple roles at the same time, even those not formally recognized. Each role comes with its own set of moral duties, which can potentially conflict with one another. In this sense, an agent is morally responsible toward their progeny (as a parent), toward other members of their community (as a citizen), toward humanity and other species (as a rational being), and, if they are a doctor, toward their patients (Magni, 2019).

According to Hart, it is controversial to consider *every* obligation deriving from occupying a particular role as a responsibility (H. L. A. Hart, 1968/2008). Slightly modifying an example from Hart, who refers to a soldier and their superior, consider a student who has duties in virtue of being a student, such as studying, attending classes, and respecting their fellow students, class, and teachers. These duties – which we may call duties-responsibilities – are part of a "sphere of responsibility", since they are relatively complex and extensive and require care or attention over an extended period of time. On the contrary, short-lived duties of a very simple kind, to do or not to do a specific act on a particular occasion, may not fall within such sphere of responsibility, e.g., fulfilling the teacher's request to close the door. These distinctions underscore the alleged importance of features such as complexity and duration for including a duty within the domain of role responsibility.

However, some authors believe there is nothing helpful in making such a distinction: every duty of a person occupying a specific role is a duty-responsibility, falling within the sphere of responsibility generated by the role an agent covers (Duff, 2007). In support of this last perspective, I argue that while it is intuitively true that a duty-responsibility is something more general and complex compared to a simple and immediate duty, compliance with the former is given by respecting the latter on an ongoing basis. For instance, by obeying a simple request from a teacher, like closing the door, one inherently respects their broader authority. This exemplifies that general, long-term duties are largely upheld by consistently fulfilling more straightforward, immediate duties. Therefore, the claim that immediate and simple duties cannot be considered within the sphere of the role responsibility should be rejected.

The third use refers to *outcome responsibility* that, like role responsibility, must be understood in normative terms: the loss of the ship and the death of many passengers are attributable to Smith, who could reasonably be blamed for these events. Vincent specifies that outcome responsibility refers to the responsibility not only for the consequences of an agent's action but also for their actions (Vincent, 2011). In this way, it is possible to use the notion of outcome responsibility not only in a consequentialist sense but also in a deontological one. Unlike role responsibility, outcome responsibility is backward-looking as it should be understood in a historical sense (Cane, 2003). In this context, responsibility is inevitably linked to the notions of praise and blame. For example, a person who has been wronged can legitimately express complaints against the person responsible for the wrongdoing. Blame can be a significant aspect of inter-personal relationships, carrying with it recognition, attention, emotional connection, and respect (Fonnesu, 2018).

The fourth type of responsibility reported in the story of Captain Smith refers to the concept of *causal responsibility*. Smith's lawyer claimed that alcohol and depression were responsible for the captain's behavior and its consequences. Unlike outcome responsibility and role responsibility, causal responsibility can be understood in descriptive terms and, like out-come responsibility, is backward-looking. In this context, responsibility is a synonym for cause. Even though being the cause of a state of affairs does not necessarily mean being morally responsible for it, the overlap between causal and outcome responsibility can lead to confusion. For instance, one could say that a storm is responsible for causing a flood without imply-ing responsibility in moral terms and, accordingly, normative terms. Thus, moral responsibility and causal responsibility do not always align. Accord-ingly, there are certain capacities an individual must have in order for it to be reasonable to attribute moral responsibility to them. This is the fifth ap-plication of the term "responsibility" that we find in Captain Smith's story, and it pertains to the concept of *capacity responsibility*. Individuals can be causally, although not morally, responsible for their behaviors if they do not possess the specific cognitive capacities necessary to be held morally accountable. Very young children, for example, can commit actions that we would consider morally problematic, yet they do not meet the require-ments for moral responsibility. Consider the case where a 5-year-old child finds their grandfather's gun and uses it to shoot and kill their little sister. It would not be appropriate to hold them morally responsible for the out-comes for which, however, they might be causally responsible. Moreover, even agents who generally possess these specific cognitive capacities can be considered causally responsible and not morally responsible for the out-comes of their actions or omissions. Consider the following example:

A terrorist places a bomb in the center of Milan, which, if exploded, would cause the death of hundreds of people. The bomb's detonator is connected to a cigarette vending machine not far from the center but out of the bomb's reach. Giorgia, unaware of this and eager to buy a pack of cigarettes, uses the vending machine, triggering the bomb's detonator and causing the death of hundreds of people.[2]

It would seem rather absurd to consider Giorgia morally responsible for the deaths caused by the detonation, even though her actions indirectly led to the explosion. Indeed, Giorgia could not foresee that through her choice to use a vending machine, she would cause a massacre, as typically, cigarette vending machines do not trigger bomb explosions. If, however, Giorgia had known that by using that vending machine she would have caused the massacre and decided to use it anyway, the moral judgment on her behavior would undoubtedly be different.[3]

In light of these considerations, we can distinguish at least three types of capacities that are essential for attributing moral responsibility to an agent: *material capacity*, *moral capacity* (also known as moral agency), and *epistemic capacity*.

The first type of capacity is that of materially causing an action or, generally speaking, a particular state of affairs. For instance, Giorgia has the capacity to use the automatic cigarette vending machine, thereby triggering the detonator,[4] and the five-year-old child has the capacity to pull the trigger of their grandfather's gun. This capacity may even be attributed to storms causing floods or electrical leakages causing fires.

The second type of capacity involves the ability to deliberate and decide how to act morally; hence, the capacity to evaluate the situation in order to make a moral decision. In the story of Captain Smith, this second type of capability comes into play: since Smith was not dealing with depression at the time of the incident, the prosecution argued that his mental capacities were unimpaired and, therefore, that his moral judgment was not compromised. In other words, Smith had full cognitive and volitional capabilities, which Hart describes as the ability to understand what we ought to do, deliberate morally, make decisions, and control our actions accordingly (H. L. A. Hart, 1968/2008). To bear moral responsibility for something, one must be a moral agent, that is, an individual capable of expressing moral judgments based on some notion of right and wrong and, consequently, acting based on reasons related to these notions.[5] Many philosophers believe that only rational individuals capable of expressing self-interested judgments can be considered moral agents. Assuming that most adult human beings possess these capacities, as in Smith's case, we can consider them morally responsible for their behaviors. In contrast, other categories – such as non-human animals, very young children, those suffering from severe developmental disabilities or dementia, those suffering from severe forms of depression or mental illnesses, and even those who temporarily lose their rational capacities – cannot be assigned, at least not in full, responsibility for their actions or omissions.[6]

By epistemic capacity, I refer to the ability to know or foresee the state of affairs that will reasonably be created in light of the agent's action or omission. It is similar to what Randolph Clarke calls the "epistemic condition", namely, the belief or awareness of what one is doing, often concerned with knowledge or awareness of the moral status as well of one's conduct (Clarke, 2022). Let us consider again the case of Giorgia and the bomb triggered by the vending machine. When activating the vending machine, Giorgia possesses both material capacity – the capacity of materially activating the machine – and moral capacity – she had the full ability to deliberate and decide how to act morally. However, she did not know that activating the vending machine would have triggered the bomb's detonator. Where consequences are improbable or unpredictable, ignorance about them generally exculpates the agent. Unintentional consequences, therefore, fall under the only domain of causal responsibility, not moral responsibility. Of course, the absence of epistemic capacity does not avoid the attribution of moral responsibility when the agent has not adequately investigated or taken seriously the probable consequences of their action or omission.[7] To stress the distinction between moral and epistemic capacity, let us review the example of Giorgia. As I have already said, if Giorgia had known that activating the vending machine would have triggered the bomb's detonator, her willingness to use it would undoubtedly have been reprehensible since, at that point, she would also possess the epistemic capacity necessary for the attribution of moral responsibility. Assuming now that the terrorist who put the bomb in the center of Milan had tricked Mark, a person with serious mental problems and paranoia, into using the vending machine, while not hiding the consequences of that act, but justifying them with bizarre speeches regarding the salvation of the world and the evil necessary for its achievement. In that case, Mark would have possessed the epistemic capacity – he knew that activating the vending machine would have triggered the bomb's detonator – but not the moral ones – he did not know how to manage information within a moral deliberation due to his mental illness.

Lastly, the sixth type of responsibility is associated with being subject to sanctions. This type of responsibility, which Hart calls *liability responsibility*, is undoubtedly central in the legal context but can also play a role in the moral realm. In Captain Smith's case, Vincent mentions the financial compensation for the harm suffered by the victims. Thus, the concept of responsibility comes into play when establishing an agent's obligation to make amends for their actions and how they should be treated during the process of remediation (Vincent, 2011).

2.1.1 Integrating the Different Types of Responsibility

Despite their different meanings, the various uses of responsibility are interconnected and should be considered in a coordinated and interrelated way. Therefore, it is necessary to highlight and, in some respects, reiterate the connections between the different ways of understanding responsibility. The primary focus will be on the notions of outcome responsibility and role responsibility, which serve as the crucial normative elements when referring to moral responsibility.

Outcome responsibility depends on the concepts of causal responsibility and role responsibility. When we deal with an event (such as Captain Smith's sunken boat and the deaths of passengers or the bomb explosion in Giorgia and the terrorist's case), as Vincent points out, the first question that needs to be addressed to determine the attribution of outcome responsibility is the following: "who was it?" (Vincent, 2011). This implies that we need to determine who (or what) bears the causal responsibility for the outcome. Clearly, in this context, I am not referring solely to the "ultimate" cause that led to a particular event, as every event is the product of a background set of contributory conditions. In fact, we should assess which actions or omissions have decisively contributed to the occurrence of a specific state of affairs.[8] Therefore, causal responsibility is a necessary condition for attributing outcome responsibility.

However, considering the previously discussed distinction between causal responsibility, a descriptive term, and moral responsibility, a normative concept, and since these concepts are not always superimposable, we can quickly notice that causal responsibility is not a sufficient element for attributing outcome responsibility. We also need to consider role responsibility: only if the causally responsible agent of the event under evaluation retrospectively acted differently or in line with how they should have acted from a moral point of view can they be considered morally responsible.

Both role responsibility and causal responsibility concepts, in turn, rely on capacity responsibility. To be causally responsible for carrying out a certain action or to bring about a certain state of affairs, an agent must have the actual capacity to produce the result under moral scrutiny (material capacity). Role responsibility instead depends on all three kinds of capacity, namely, material, moral, and epistemic. This relationship encapsulates the idea that the moral duty to perform or refrain from an action implies the capacity to do so. Since Immanuel Kant was the paradigmatic proponent of this notion, this argument is often called "Kantian". Kant argued that an agent has a moral obligation to perform (or not perform) an action only if they have the capacity to perform (or not perform) that action. He says, "The action to which the 'ought' applies must indeed be possible under natural conditions" (Kant, 1781/1929, p. 473). In essence, "ought implies can". This argument holds validity not only in moral contexts but also in legal ones, an instance of what is frequently referred to with the Latin maxim *ad impossibilia nemo tenetur*. However, the Kantian principle can bear different interpretations, contingent on the meaning attributed to "can".[9] This is particularly relevant with regard to material capacity, for which "can" can be defined not only in terms of what is physically possible for the agent or in accordance with the laws of nature but also, more specifically, in technological terms – a topic I will discuss in the subsequent section.[10]

2.1.2 *Procreative Responsibility as Role Responsibility*

In light of the taxonomy presented and the relationship between the different concepts of responsibility, I can conclude that the concept of procreative responsibility I have in mind in this work should be understood primarily as a kind of role responsibility. Thus, the following pages aim to evaluate – from a forward-looking perspective – whether there are – and, if so, which – moral obligations or duties an individual faces as they play the role of procreator in the field of the continuous development of assisted reproduction technologies. Certainly, given the connection between the various kinds of responsibility that we have seen, I will sometimes refer to outcome responsibility, specifically when I discuss legitimate complaints against procreators by those affected by a specific procreative choice. This discussion presupposes that procreators have a certain causal responsibility for the state of affairs generated by the procreative choice. Nonetheless, procreative responsibility as role responsibility remains the main focus of this work.

2.2   Material Capacity and Technological Development

If role responsibility depends on the agent's material capabilities, procreative responsibility as role responsibility will depend on the material capabilities of the procreator. An agent's material capacity is not solely based on internal factors, namely, their cognitive or physical abilities, but also based on their ability to control external factors. Technological conditions, which can be understood as tools enabling the agent to carry out certain actions, belong to this category.[11] Therefore, the question arises as to how to interpret the development of technological conditions in light of moral responsibility.

Generally, what belongs to the domain of nature is understood as a given fact and as something that cannot be framed in terms of moral responsibility (Buchanan et al., 2000). Based on this viewpoint, human conditions that are dependent on natural factors, like having a genetic disease, are often seen in terms of luck, misfortune, or, more generally, chance. This is because what belongs to the domain of nature is outside human control. In light of what has been said in the previous sections, it seems implausible to define in moral terms something that does not depend on the material capacity of the human being. However, the limits of what we describe as "natural" are not at all static (Bayertz, 2003), especially in the field of medical and technological development. The bioethical enterprise was born in light of the need for new reflection in the face of biomedicine, that of the second half of the 20th century, now oriented in a scientific and experimental sense and increasingly supported by new technological intervention tools.

In this context, technological development is frequently perceived as a tool that expands the range of available options. The bioethical reflection of the first decades was indeed primarily focused on normatively evaluating the *permissibility* of medical practices made possible thanks to technological development, such as organ transplantation and assisted reproduction.[12] Notwithstanding, technology enhances human control over occurrences that previously belonged to the realm of nature. In other words, we face an expansion of the material capacity of moral agents. If it is true that material capacities determine which role responsibilities can be attributed to an agent, then this means that technology can modify the extent of moral obligations toward others (Swierstra & Waelbers, 2012). Indeed, by altering or expanding our options, technology "mediates" our (moral) reasons for action, thereby extending our responsibility (Waelbers, 2011).[13] In a nutshell, our moral obligations are deeply dependent on what we can control.[14]

According to Allen Buchanan and colleagues, what is generally considered "moral progress" historically involves pushing back the boundaries of the natural, bringing into the realm of human control, and thus into the domain of justice and ethics, what was previously considered natural and hence merely a matter of good or bad luck.[15] The authors observe that "[p]aradoxically, nature brought within human control is no longer nature" (Buchanan et al., 2000, p. 83). In the field of medicine, this argument can be presented with a rather familiar scenario, an attitude generally accepted, at least in certain contexts, by common-sense morality. Consider, for instance, a doctor treating a patient with pancreatic cancer, a condition for which no cure exists. Given the doctor's material inability to treat the patient's disease, their duty to the patient is limited to palliative care, intended to alleviate the patient's suffering in their final moments. However, should advancements in scientific and technological knowledge produce an effective cure for pancreatic cancer available to the doctor, the doctor would be expected to treat the patient with it. Failing to do so could render them morally (and likely legally) responsible for the patient's death.[16]

2.2.1   The Colonization of Reproduction by Ethics

The aforementioned argument can also be applied to human reproduction. The technological developments of recent decades and the increased quality of life in Western societies indeed provide reasons to discuss a possible extension to the boundaries of procreative responsibility (Buchanan et al.,

2000). Thanks to ARTs, as introduced in the first chapter, many aspects of reproduction no longer fall within the scope of a natural process outside human control, but within the realm of what we can control.

From this perspective, John Rawls's distinction between natural and social goods may blur (Del Bò, 2004; Loi, 2010), as some phenotypic traits of the future individual may effectively become a social product, dependent on cultural and institutional factors (Farrelly, 2002), and even on parental choices. Paraphrasing Buchanan and colleagues, this would then inaugurate *a colonization of human reproduction by ethics* (Buchanan et al., 2000, p. 45). The new possibilities of biotechnological intervention could, therefore, imply an expansion of procreators' responsibility.

Unlike the example of the doctor and the pancreatic cancer cure mentioned previously, however, when this argument is applied to human reproduction, it appears to conflict with many people's moral intuitions. Indeed, historical understanding views current techniques as tools for enhancing future parents' reproductive freedom (Davis, 1997), not as a means to broaden their responsibilities. This perspective partly stems from the emphasis nowadays society puts on the private nature of human reproduction (Davis, 2010), the emotional implications, and the notable correlation between the possibility of early-life genetic interventions and contentious eugenic theories (Battisti, 2019).

2.3   Responsibility, Parenting, Procreation, and Reproduction

In line with Buchanan and colleagues, some bioethicists have proposed models or principles to balance the claims of reproductive freedom or autonomy – the principle that competent members of society would have the right to freely choose how, when, and where to reproduce (Robertson, 1994) – with those related to procreative responsibility (Buller & Bauer, 2011). I call these "models of procreative responsibility" or "principles of procreative responsibility". Future chapters will address these principles, examining their specific content and alleged justifications. In this section, however, I aim to establish a formal definition of procreative responsibility. This analysis is essential for a more comprehensive understanding of the various models of procreative responsibility proposed in the literature, as well as their application to the continually evolving field of ARTs.

To understand the relationship between the definition of procreative responsibility and its various models, it may be useful to draw on a distinction suggested by Rawls (2009) between "concept" and "conception". A concept identifies the basic semantic element of a particular word, while a conception is a specific normative proposal related to that concept. Due to its general and abstract nature, a broad consensus can be formed around a concept, even among those who hold differing conceptions of it.

The concept, therefore, forms the analytical backbone of moral discourse to the various conceptions. Thus, if the definition of procreative responsibility that I will present below pertains to the concept, the models or principles of procreative responsibility will relate to the different conceptions one can adopt. It is important to note that while a broader consensus might be achieved around the concept compared to the conceptions, this does not imply that a consensus on a specific conception of procreative responsibility is unattainable. The aim of the subsequent chapters is precisely to propose a conception that can be embraced from various moral standpoints.[17]

To define the concept of procreative responsibility, I will first analyze the less obscure concept of parental responsibility, also presenting the conception that seems to be rather shared in contemporary Western societies. Then, I investigate the relationship between parental responsibility and responsibility in the procreative context. As we have seen, the general concept of responsibility is quite ambiguous, perhaps even more so in the context of human reproduction. To refer to the notion of responsibility in the reproductive context, the terms "procreative responsibility", "reproductive responsibility", and "parental responsibility" are often used interchangeably. However, I propose that these terms should not be considered synonyms and will suggest a helpful distinction.

2.3.1 Parental Responsibility

Broadly speaking, parental responsibility can be understood as the obligations parents have toward their children. Parental responsibility is described here in terms of role responsibility, and it suggests that parents have a unique relationship with their children, unlike non-parents. This unique relationship is characterized by the particularistic care that parents should provide to their specific children (Overall, 2012).

Societal, cultural, and scientific developments constantly shape and shift the boundaries of parental responsibility. While in today's Western societies, children are generally seen as bearers of rights and vulnerable members of our societies requiring additional protections compared to adults, this trend is relatively recent (Archard, 2014). In the past, children were often viewed as parents' property and a source of cheap labor (Pinchbeck & Hewitt, 1973; S. N. Hart, 1991). However, in the last century, discussions around parental responsibility and shared perceptions of children's moral status and their place in family and society have allowed us to recognize not only parental rights over children, as was previously the case, but also duties toward offspring (Gheaus, 2012).[18] The UK's Law Commission has even argued that discussing matters related to the relationship between parents and children should be framed in terms of parental responsibility, deeming the concept of parental rights over children inappropriate, both legally and colloquially (UK Law Commission, 1982). As Kriestien Hens and colleagues observe, parents are now reasonably held accountable for their children's cognitive and socio-emotional development; hence, parental obligations toward their offspring are not only limited to providing children with a home, feeding them, taking them to the doctor when they fall ill, and sending them to school (Hens et al., 2017). Furthermore, some argue that parents are also responsible for their children's physical development and should thus prevent the onset of obesity in their offspring (Holm, 2008).

A central aspect of contemporary parental responsibility undoubtedly relates to medical decisions for the child. In this context, the principle of "child's best interest" has been introduced, and it is the parents' responsibility to ensure its fulfillment, given their ability to provide care (Bridgeman, 2007). The concept of the child's best interest is complex and can sometimes cause conflict between healthcare professionals and parents, or even among parents themselves[19]; generally, in the medical context, a parent acts in the child's best interest when they prioritize the child's interests over their own when choosing treatments and care (Bester, 2019).

More generally, it is widely accepted that parents should promote their children's future autonomy and self-realization. This idea was primarily put forth by Joel Feinberg in his article "The Child's Right to an Open Future" (Feinberg, 1980). According to Feinberg, there are two types of "C-Rights" or rights that belong only to children: on the one hand, "dependency rights",[20] which derive from a child's dependence on others for basic life goods such as food, housing, and protection; and on the other, "rights in trust", namely, child rights that must be preserved until they become adults. The child is not yet capable of exercising such rights; therefore, they should be protected so that the child, once an adult, has the opportunity to exercise them. Although rights in trust are a heterogeneous set, they fall within the broader category of "right to an open future" or "anticipatory autonomy right". This refers to all rights attributable to adult persons but must be safeguarded during childhood to be exercisable in the future.

An example of a right that falls within the child's right to an open future is the right to reproduce (Cutas & Hens, 2015).[21] As children are not physically capable of reproducing, they cannot exercise this right currently. However, once grown, the individual will be able to exercise such a right (Davis, 2010). Therefore, in order to have the opportunity to exercise their procreative rights, a child has the right not to be sterilized by their parents. To sum up, Feinberg argues that parents should ensure that "basic options are kept open and growth kept natural or unforced" (Feinberg, 1980, p. 127).[22]

It is outside the scope of this work to provide a strong defense of such a conception of parental responsibility. I limit myself to arguing that the idea of a parent meeting the aforementioned child's needs aligns with many people's considered moral judgments, especially in Western societies. This provides a robust starting point for analyzing the more complex concept of responsibility in the reproductive context.

2.3.2 Procreative Responsibility

It is not always clear which kinds of duties or obligations fall within procreative responsibility. In some reproductive contexts, procreative responsibility may coincide with parental responsibility. From this perspective, the question "what do we owe to our children?" should be asked not only after the child's birth but also before it (DeGrazia, 2016). In other words, the moral duties of procreators should be considered within the broader realm of parental responsibility, thus recognizing a continuity between these responsibilities. The procreator, considered in every sense already a parent, should be guided at least by some of the moral reasons that would guide them in the relationship with already existing children.[23] For clarity, here I introduce the concept of *procreative-parental responsibility*, which consists of the set of moral duties of the procreator as a future parent.

According to some bioethicists, however, the moral obligations of those who generate new individuals should not be limited to the ones that fall within the scope of procreative-parental responsibility but should also be extended in relation to individuals who are outside the parent–child relationship. From this perspective, procreation could significantly impact an already existing child of the procreator, the family in the broader sense, or even society. Indeed, generating a child with certain characteristics (Anomaly, 2014, 2018; Brock, 2005) or generating more children without considering the problem of overpopulation also related to environmental concerns (Cafaro, 2012; Das Gupta, 2014; Häyry, 2023; Hickey et al., 2016; Vance, 2024) could have an impact on social welfare or on the rights of other people, which should not be neglected in reproductive choice (Cavaliere, 2020). In this context, we can refer to a distinction already proposed by David Wasserman that provocatively distinguishes the role of the parent, who must take care of the child who will be born, and that of the progenitor, who would be a sort of gatekeeper in the service of the interests of family or society in which the future individual will grow (Wasserman, 2005). Thus, we can differentiate between procreative responsibility and procreative-parental responsibility, a distinction that, although seldom explicit, plays a central role in discussions around procreative responsibility models and their moral justifications.[24]

In light of this first distinction, I propose a more specific taxonomy to clarify the concept of responsibility in the context of procreation. I define procreative responsibility as the set of moral obligations or duties of procreators in general terms. Within procreative responsibility, two subcategories are observed. The first subcategory is the aforementioned procreative-parental responsibility. In this context, the moral question that procreators ask themselves should be the same as what they ask once the child is born. However, it is evident that procreative-parental responsibility in the procreative context is only a part of the broader definition of parental responsibility. This broader responsibility involves moral duties toward children. These duties extend beyond the act of procreation and continue after they are born.

Procreative responsibility also includes requests that fall within the label *reproductive responsibility*, that is, the set of moral obligations that an individual has as a mere reproducer. In this context, reproducers must ask themselves: "What effect will my reproductive act have on others or, more generally, on the world?". Reproductive responsibility thus extends beyond the direct parent–child bond, encompassing broader ethical considerations in a series of expanding moral circles, each representing varying degrees of impact on individuals affected by the act of procreation. We can identify at least three types of reproductive responsibility: *parental-reproductive responsibility* has to do with the set of moral obligations that reproducers have toward their existing children. *Family-based reproductive responsibility* concerns reproducers' moral obligations toward their own family unit. *Broad reproductive responsibility* involves duties toward society and the world at large.

In addition, a further distinction can be recognized within the domain of reproductive responsibility, which intersects the categories mentioned previously. This distinction is based on the orientation of the responsibility: *quality-oriented reproductive responsibility* arises when prospective parents are faced with the decision to procreate a child with specific characteristics, achieved through either embryo selection or genetic modification via reproductive Genome Editing (rGE) or other techniques. *Quantity-oriented reproductive responsibility*, conversely, involves the consideration of limiting the number of children to prevent negative impacts on other existing children, family members, or society due to concerns about overpopulation.

In this work, I thus differentiate between the often-interchangeable terms "reproductive responsibility" and "procreative responsibility". Some may reject the term "procreation" to secularize the bioethical vocabulary (Mori, 2020). Indeed, while the term "procreation" derives from the Latin word *procreatio*, meaning "creating on behalf of" and has been predominantly used in theological contexts, "reproduction" refers to the act or process of reproducing and is used scientifically to describe human, animal, and cellular reproduction. Despite my work being committed to an eminently secular perspective, I do not reject the term "procreation"; instead, I attribute to it a new meaning, more general and different from the more specific term "reproduction". The latter indicates only the reproductive act and its effects, while I will use the former term more broadly: it will also indicate the existence of a relationship between the future parent and the future child.

In summary, procreative responsibility is a broader concept that encompasses reproductive responsibility but is not limited to it. It can also include uniquely procreative-parental aspects. As already said in the introduction, I will focus mainly on procreative-parental responsibility, although some considerations relating to reproductive responsibility will still be proposed. With regard to the latter, it is important to note that discussing reproductive responsibility, particularly in terms of broad reproductive responsibility, can be particularly controversial. Indeed, the existence of moral duties in merely reproductive terms directly echoes some eugenics claims, not so much in its liberal version – where reproductive interventions are private in nature and, therefore, subordinate to the preferences of the reproducer and, in the more moderate versions, also to the interests of the future individual – but in the classical version, which pursued the goal of creating a better society and maintaining a specific genetic pool (Battisti, 2019; Buchanan et al., 2000; Cavaliere, 2018; Wikler, 1999). However, proponents of these new duties do not advocate a form of state-promoted coercive eugenics; on the contrary, according to them, it might be desirable to promote education on genetics and assisted reproduction techniques so that procreators can make autonomous and aware choices, for example, on the desired traits of future children (Anomaly, 2018). In this context, in fact, procreative freedom is not denied but viewed as an imperfect yet essential tool to deal with procreative decisions (Cavaliere, 2020).[25]

2.3.3   How Should Procreative Responsibility Be Understood?

Thanks to the proposed taxonomy, I have introduced concepts that will guide us in the discussion concerning procreative responsibility models, introducing different kinds of duties that people may face when they decide to reproduce. However, it should be reiterated that I have not yet provided any moral justification for the existence of such duties: for instance, while I have set forth the notion of procreative-parental responsibility as the set of duties a procreator has as a parent, I have not yet offered any moral justification or argument for the existence of this duties. In other words, at this juncture, without any justification, the kinds of duties classified within the aforementioned taxonomy remain putative. But before I delve into the intricacies of procreative responsibility and explore the various models highlighted in the literature, it is crucial to set the context. While some might think these new moral duties must be strictly observed if they exist, I argue this is not the proper way to interpret procreative responsibility. It is at least doubtful that any moral principle or duty, understood not in simplistic and trivial terms, is so strong (Savulescu & Kahane, 2009b). Moreover, considering procreative obligations as absolute overlooks the morally complex nature of human reproduction and the experience of parenthood. Other morally relevant factors can play an essential role in informing procreative choices. This might contrast with certain procreative duties and, accordingly, reduce the normative force of prescriptions relating to procreative responsibility.

Human reproduction encompasses psychological and social aspects, which can cause significant burdens, especially for women and people with the capacity to become pregnant, and cannot be neglected in the moral choices we will discuss in this work. For instance, considerable pressure often accompanies deciding "when" to have a child, a choice heavily influenced by family, friends, acquaintances, and broader societal norms (Bergnéhr, 2009). Furthermore, it is known that the decision to procreate can be characterized by the emergence of various concerns and fears related, for example, to the future stability of the relationship between the parents, the commitment that one or more children can involve, or the fear of not being a good parent. Miscarriages and, more generally, reproductive losses occurring during the attempt to have a child could cause significant emotional stress, which could weigh on future pregnancy plans (Diamond & Diamond, 2017). Furthermore, some couples or single procreators may have economic concerns related to the procreative project, which, according to recent studies, would also have negative effects on the health of the future child (A. M. Mitchell & Christian, 2017). In addition to these considerations, it is important to remember the physical burdens often endured by pregnant people during pregnancy.

The complexity of the procreative field is even more evident when we consider the ongoing development of ARTs. As already observed in Chapter 1, techniques such as *In Vitro* Fertilization and Preimplantation Genetic Diagnosis (PGD) involve additional physical and psychological burdens, but this reasoning can also be extended to other techniques, including those that could be available in the future, such as rGE and ectogenesis. Despite the assumed reliability and safety of these techniques, they still carry physical and emotional burdens, particularly for pregnant people. Moreover, other relevant factors potentially causing anxiety and distress should be considered. For example, genomic knowledge combined with the use of reproductive techniques could generate new psychological burdens: acquiring information on the genome of the future individual could lead to the discovery of genetic predispositions in the parents themselves, who would have preferred not to know their own conditions (Anderson et al., 2017). In this regard, think of a parent who, through DNA analysis of the embryo before transfer to the uterus, discovers that they carry genetic variants associated with autism, cancer, schizophrenia, or early Alzheimer's disease (Flatau et al., 2018).[26]

Moreover, the new moral duties that could emerge from the development of ARTs could clash with parents' identities and values. If parents oppose these practices, they may face pressure and significant psychological distress. In this line, Josephine Johnston – critically discussing the moral duties that the availability of the genome editing technique could bring out – argues that some parents would not want to conceive of themselves as the "maker" or "fixer" of their future children (Johnston, 2019). Moreover, others could argue that reproduction techniques such as ectogenesis would have effects on the way some parents conceive of parenthood and the relationship with the future child. According to this perspective, the symbolic value of the experience of conception and pregnancy would be radically disrupted.

Based on these reasons, I argue that procreative responsibility prescriptions should be *prima facie* ones.[27] In other words, while these reasons, duties, or obligations warrant serious consideration, they are not absolute.[28] Rather, they should be weighed against other morally relevant considerations, as previously discussed. Furthermore, understanding the requests of procreative responsibility in *prima facie* terms makes these reflections compatible with a permissive legislative context regarding procreative choices. This, in turn, is compatible with a framework that condemns any coercive act based on new moral duties linked to the procreative sphere. This approach allows us to refute criticisms asserting that exploring new moral responsibilities of parents necessarily overlooks the importance of procreative freedom and the complexity of human reproduction. Moreover, this also allows us not to ignore the basic feminist principle of concern for women's well-being and reproductive rights (Overall, 2012), bearing in mind that these considerations can be extended to all pregnant people.

However, these aspects should not be used as a pretext to dismiss technological development as a sufficient reason to at least contemplate the emergence of new forms of procreative responsibility. In opposite direction, Vincent and Emma A. Jane argue that future parents already face substantial pressures, suggesting that adding further responsibilities may be excessive (Vincent & Jane, 2019). In other words, parents may be unable to sustain the emotional strain of new moral obligations. According to the authors, this is even more evident if one considers the possible social pressure that future parents could undergo to use certain reproductive technologies in light of their availability and diffusion.

Regarding procreative choices, it is vital to balance the interests of future parents and the consequences for future individuals and society (Johnston, 2019). However, this does not mean that the interests of parents should always take precedence. Furthermore, authors who argue that new moral obligations could cause psychological overload must acknowledge that this viewpoint is not neutral; it is heavily influenced by historical and cultural contexts. This argument stems from a model of parenthood and procreation that is well contextualized in history and culture. In the future, our current understanding of the emerging procreative context could become normalized. This normalization might bring changes – not necessarily negative – in our understanding of parenthood from moral, psychological, and social perspectives. In other words, using the argument of excessive physical and emotional load to avoid considering the new and emerging requests of procreative responsibility is inappropriate. Even if we admit the relevance of these aspects, they cannot diminish the significance of moral reasons connected to procreative responsibility, which emerge from new reproductive scenarios. Clearly, such new reasons will then always have to be balanced with the considerations about reproduction described above. However, this can occur appropriately only after such reasons have been clearly identified and investigated.

I acknowledge the significant impact new reproductive technologies could have on the procreative choices of prospective parents. However, even in this case, this should not preclude the possibility of reflecting on the redefinition of the boundaries of procreative responsibility. Ethical reasoning, understood as a critical, autonomous, and non-dogmatic reflection on our moral judgments and – broadly speaking – moral systems, becomes a valuable tool in this context. For example, it can help prospective parents navigate societal pressures favoring certain procreative choices. From this perspective, reasoning about procreative responsibility can certainly help prospective parents understand the morally relevant aspects at stake and, accordingly, make informed choices.

2.4   Procreative Responsibility and Disability

In the previous sections, I argued that procreative and parental obligations could depend on what is referred to as material capacity. However, they also rely on another aspect, which is undoubtedly controversial: the definition of disability prospective parents endorse.

It is generally considered one of the parents' moral duties to prevent or, at the very least, minimize disabilities in their child's life. As will be more explicit in the following chapters, there are good reasons to believe such duties should also be extended to some procreative contexts. Nevertheless, there is a crucial aspect that needs to be made explicit here: a necessary, albeit not sufficient, condition for attributing a moral obligation to avoid certain conditions in offspring is to recognize those conditions as a form of disability or, in any case, that these conditions are negative for the affected individual or, more generally, for the world.

There is significant disagreement about the meaning of the concept of disability, also in light of the structural discriminations that people with disabilities have suffered in the past and still suffer today. For instance, a 2018 study states that people with disabilities, especially mental ones, report a perception of a higher degree of violence and discrimination against them compared to individuals not affected by disabilities (Dammeyer & Chapman, 2018). This aspect is even more evident if we consider the aforementioned eugenic practices, in particular those that took place in Nazi Germany, which involved the systematic sterilization and extermination of individuals with certain forms of disabilities (D. Mitchell & Snyder, 2003).

Moreover, some bioethicists and disability rights movements have argued that the increase and development of selective practices at the beginning of life were sources of further discrimination (Hofmann, 2017; Wise, 2012). This is known as the "expressivist" argument or objection (Parens & Asch, 2003; Wendell, 1996); it posits that opting for biotechnological techniques to treat or prevent the birth of individuals with certain traits undermines the value of existing individuals who already possess these traits. Through the use of prenatal genetic tests to select a "healthy" embryo or the decision to abort a fetus with malformations or specific genetic conditions, prospective parents or, more broadly, society would express a negative judgment about people with disabilities, thereby denying the equality of moral dignity among people. The idea is that genetic selection through PGD and prenatal diagnosis techniques implies that the lives of people with disabilities are not worth living and, therefore, are intrinsically discriminatory.

While the expressivist argument is invoked against the possibility of allowing people to freely decide whether or not to have a child with some disability, it is advanced even more strongly against those who argue in favor of the existence of moral duties to make procreative choices that avoid certain forms of disability (Bennett, 2009). The expressivist argument is complex and will not be expanded upon in this work as it deserves its own detailed discussion. However, as noted by disability rights scholar and activist Thomas Shakespeare, it is worth mentioning that recognizing and promoting the rights of people with disabilities is not at odds with "curing" or "treating" these conditions (Shakespeare, 2014). They could even be viewed as complementary approaches. Any further consideration about disability in the procreative context, however, depends on its definition. In the following sections, I will elaborate on four different definitions provided within the ongoing debate on disability.

2.4.1 The Medical Model

The Medical Model of Disability considers disability as the presence of long-lasting physical, mental, intellectual, or sensory impairments that lead to the loss of the normal functioning of the human species. This model is also called "individual" because it tends to conceive disability as primarily, if not solely, related to the bearers of the condition (Rothman, 2010). Therefore, the Medical Model is based on a comparison with norms and standards that define the functioning of human beings (Boorse, 1982). For example, there is a norm for sight and gradations of poor vision that ultimately leads to total loss of sight or blindness. People who deviate from the norm and who cannot be made functional according to the norm through assistive devices, surgery, treatments, or other means are considered "disabled" (Rothman, 2018).

John Harris criticized this model, noting that people can be "normal" and still be disabled in some sense. Suppose that, due to further depletions of the ozone layer, all white-skinned people are very vulnerable to skin cancers even with slight sun exposure, but dark and black-skinned people are immune. According to Harris, people with white pigmentation are essentially disabled compared to people with darker skin. And if skin pigmentation could be easily altered, the failure to make alterations would be disabling. Harris thus argues that disability is the kind of harmed condition in which a person has a rational preference not to be, and the definition of this condition does not depend on what is the normal functioning of the species (Harris, 2001). The definition of a "harmed condition" is certainly controversial. Some have argued that a harmed condition largely depends on the social context in which people with certain characteristics find themselves. The most radical defense of this thesis is supported by proponents of the Social Model of Disability.

2.4.2 The Social Model

The Social Model of Disability – historically strongly asserted by movements for the rights of people with disabilities (Shakespeare, 2017) – argues that people with disabilities find themselves in damaged and oppressed conditions not so much because they possess characteristics that deviate from the normal functioning of the species, but because of the existence of systemic barriers, contemptuous attitudes, and social exclusion (intentional or unintentional), which harm people affected by certain conditions. In other words, the social context determines the "harmed situation" that some individuals are in. The Social Model of Disability thus departs from the Medical Model: although physical, sensory, intellectual, or psychological variations may cause individual functional limitations or impairments, these would not necessarily lead to a disability, unless society fails to consider and include people regardless of their individual differences. In this context, disability is understood not as an "individual" aspect but as a public issue. The Social Model of Disability also defines people with disabilities as a minority, a group oppressed by dominant classes in society. As the Union of the Physically Impaired Against Segregation argued:

> In our view, it is society which disables physically impaired people. Disability is something imposed on top of our impairments by the way we are unnecessarily isolated and excluded from full participation in society. Disabled people are therefore an oppressed group in society.
>
> (1976, p. 4)

The Social Model has been very successful in the last 50 years; in fact, it has been politically effective and has enabled the construction of a social movement of people with disabilities (Hasler, 1993). This movement contributed to the effective identification of social barriers that did not allow equal access opportunities for people with disabilities and to the promotion of self-esteem for people with these conditions (Shakespeare, 2014).

However, as several experts in so-called disability studies recognize, the Social Model lends itself to numerous criticisms. First, by strongly rejecting individual and medical approaches, it risks conceiving impairment as something non-problematic, and thus neglects the experience and the relationship between the individual and their own condition (Crow, 1992).

Second, according to Shakespeare, the Social Model assumes what it needs to prove. In its definition, it states that disability is a condition of oppression. In other words, what is at stake is not whether disabled people are oppressed in a particular situation but only the extent to which they are oppressed. In this circular perspective, it becomes logically impossible to observe people with disabilities who are not oppressed (Shakespeare, 2014).

Third, the Social Model seems to implicitly lead not only to the guarantee of civil rights for people with disabilities but also to a proper "right to disability". People with certain conditions could exercise this putative right in choosing certain traits for their offspring both in the reproductive context and after the birth of their children. Many people with impairments, consistent with the Social Model, do not perceive their condition as a source of disability. For example, both deafness and achondroplastic short stature have been understood as cultural traits, rather than disabling conditions, by many individuals who have them and by many disability rights movements. The logical step that this model allows is that the choice to deliberately conceive a child with a disability should be a right for prospective parents (Benston, 2016; Camporesi, 2010).

2.4.3   *The Welfarist Model*

The first alternative model to the ones presented above is the Welfarist Model, proposed by Julian Savulescu and Guy Kahane (Savulescu & Kahane, 2009a, 2011). According to its proponents, this approach incorporates insights from both the Medical and Social Models, leaving aside their more implausible aspects. Like the Social Model, the welfare approach denies that the human species' normal functioning is morally significant. Like the Medical Model, it does not consider social prejudice the only source of the resulting associated disadvantage. According to the Welfarist Model, the concept of disability refers to any stable physical or psychological property of a subject S that leads to a significant reduction in their level of well-being in circumstances C. Notice, however, the effect this condition has on well-being due to social prejudice toward S by members of S's society is excluded (Savulescu & Kahane, 2011). The authors argue that the Social Model is correct in claiming that adverse effects of deviation from the species norm are due to such prejudice. However, they point out that this does not imply that *all* of the ways in which typical disabilities can negatively affect well-being are *entirely* due to prejudice.

Moreover, unlike the Medical Model, the Welfarist Model makes no reference to the biostatistical definition of "normality" or health, but uses a normative tool, namely, the concept of well-being: if a property in certain circumstances C produces a reduction in well-being for a person, then this condition is negative for this person. Disability, therefore, depends on the context and circumstances. What makes it harder to lead a good life in one particular circumstance may make it easier in another.

However, this model does not intend to provide specific tools to fight disability, which could be resolved either through a change in a person's biology, as the Medical Model suggests, or through a change in society, as the Social Model suggests. In this case, the answer changes depending on potential treatments' costs, efficacy, and safety. In other words, it does not argue that disadvantages caused by disability should be tackled only through the breaking down of social barriers, but it affirms a certain neutrality toward the means by which this end is pursued.

Note that the Welfarist Model may often lean toward the promotion of medical treatments to tackle disability rather than focusing solely on breaking down social and natural barriers, as the Social Model argues. Indeed, despite efforts to ensure an inclusive society, many people with disabilities continue to have limitations: as Shakespeare notes (2014), mountains, marshes, and beaches are almost impossible to cross for wheelchair users, while sunsets, the song of birds, and other aspects of nature are impossible to experience in the same way for those who are blind and deaf. Moreover, although many barriers can be mitigated in urban environments, historic buildings often cannot be easily adapted. Furthermore, buildings might be incompatible with barrier reduction and increased accessibility because people with different disabilities may require different solutions: people who are blind prefer defined steps and curbs and grooved pavements, while wheelchair users need ramps, lowered curbs, and smooth surfaces. The issue would become even more complex when talking about barriers for people with mental deficits and learning disabilities (Shakespeare, 2014).

According to the Welfarist Model, all people can have mild or less mild forms of disability, which always depend on the circumstances in which a person finds themselves. From this framework, two considerations emerge. The first is that dyslexia, asthma, and other conditions of this magnitude must be conceived as mild disabilities, as they diminish the well-being of carriers; this makes all people potentially affected by some form of disability. The second consideration is that even though some people have traits that, in specific conditions, reduce well-being, it may be that in other particular circumstances, these traits do not constitute a disability but rather a trait that benefits the carrier (Mills, 2011).

To better understand the Welfarist Model, it is worth reporting a widely discussed example in the bioethical debate, namely, that of the already mentioned deafness. There is indeed significant disagreement over whether deafness can be considered a disability.[29] The exemplary case is that of Sharon Duchesneau and Candy McCullough, a non-hearing couple who, in 2001, had a son named Gauvin. Sharon and Candy, both non-hearing, wanted a child who shared their common characteristic. Therefore, they decided to undergo artificial insemination using the sperm of a friend whom they knew had a family composed of non-hearing people for at least five generations. In some public statements, the couple argued that deafness is an identity, not a disability or disease that needs to be fixed or avoided.[30]

The Welfarist Model acknowledges that, generally, deafness might be understood as a disability. First, it prevents access to the world of sound: a deaf person cannot hear music, the human voice, or auditory alarms. It is true that when studying in a library, deafness is not a disability and can even be an advantageous trait; but, the ability to hear is obviously a necessary condition to enjoy those experiences that are auditory in nature. Although hearing is not a necessary characteristic for interacting with other people, without this capacity it is significantly more difficult to move in the world, respond to emergencies in which auditory alarms are present, and so on. However, the Welfarist Model does not deny a case, mostly theoretical, in which deafness could be understood as an advantage in some particular, albeit limited circumstances. This means we cannot define a biological or psychological trait, such as deafness, as a disability, since it depends on the circumstances.[31]

2.4.4 *The Equal Opportunities Model*

The second alternative model, similar to the Welfarist Model in some ways, is the Equal Opportunities Model. We can find a systematization of such a model, even if not with this name, in the famous article by Buchanan "Choosing Who Will Be Disabled: Genetic Intervention and the Morality of Inclusion" (1996). This model focuses precisely on the diminishing of equal opportunities. Although having equal opportunities also depends on having a certain degree of well-being and vice versa, this model tends to value more having access to equal opportunities to pursue one's plan for a good life. It does not, therefore, need to engage in complicated definitions of well-being, a complex and controversial concept.

Shifting the focus from well-being to opportunities allows us to consider a limitation of the Welfarist Model. An individual might have very high well-being if they lived in a specific and limited environment or under certain circumstances, even if they did not have access to equal opportunities outside this limited context. Consider, for example, the case of deafness: a person affected by deafness could enjoy high well-being if they lived in a community where sign language was known and practiced, schools were specialized in teaching non-hearing children, and deaf people held social positions and roles. However, the life plans that such an individual could pursue would primarily be limited to life within this particular community; under other circumstances, the individual would not have a range of opportunities available compared to a hearing individual. To have uncompromised well-being, the individual would be limited to a specific context, and this could, in some cases, compromise the individual's freedom to pursue their own plan for a good life.

Therefore, disability is understood here not only as the experience of physical or psychological suffering but also as a limitation of opportunities. In this context, according to Buchanan, a condition of limitation of opportunities is undesirable by definition, even if it does not involve any psycho-physical suffering (Buchanan, 1996). Disability is understood as a disadvantage. This means that disability depends not only on specific circumstances but also on the possibility of accessing a reasonable range of opportunities, that is, the suitable conditions to seek their own life plan.

According to the Equal Opportunities Model, disability is relative to the ability to perform certain specific functions, so it is wrong to talk about "disabled people", an expression nowadays even considered offensive; it is more appropriate, instead, to speak of "people with disabilities" in relation to specific functions. A person could indeed have a disability in certain areas but be able to perform other functions. More analytically, one can talk about disability when (a) a person P is not able to perform a certain function X, that is, when there is an inability to perform X; (b) the individuals in the group that P is part of can perform X[32]; and (c) the impossibility of performing X is not due to a lack of tools or knowledge of P.

Buchanan believes that each society is regulated by what he calls the "dominant cooperative framework" or "dominant cooperative scheme", the set of basic institutions and practices that allow individuals and groups to engage in mutually beneficial cooperation (Buchanan, 1996; Buchanan et al., 2000). Successfully participating in such mutually beneficial cooperation allows people to have equal opportunities within a society, meaning to have access to a reasonable number of careers, life plans, and social positions that would not be achievable outside this system. An individual will be able to participate successfully in the interaction if there is a match between their abilities and the needs of the form of interaction (Buchanan, 1996). For this reason, choosing the rules of the dominant cooperative scheme determines who will be disabled in society; therefore, selecting these rules is a matter of justice.

It is possible to identify a substantial difference between the Equal Opportunities Model and the Social Model here: according to Buchanan, the rules cannot be as inclusive as possible. The Social Model believes that social barriers are the source of the injustice that oppresses people with disabilities. However, this line of thought does not consider another legitimate interest, namely, that of non-disabled people to preserve an efficient dominant scheme.

Buchanan asks us to consider the dominant cooperative scheme of society as a card game: the people who participate can have a series of experiences such as winning, losing, having fun, and talking to other players. To give people the chance to play and enjoy the aforementioned experiences, it is first necessary to decide what card game to play and with what rules.[33] In this context, people or social groups with different abilities will legitimately advance different preferences: someone might prefer to play Bridge, a complex game, while others, such as the younger ones, who do not have the cognitive abilities to play this card game, would prefer a simpler one. While deciding to play the easier game might include the younger ones, this choice might not satisfy the people who want to play Bridge, who would have a legitimate interest in keeping the rules of the more difficult game. In this context, two legitimate sets of reasons are therefore in contrast: the reasons of people with disability to make society as inclusive as possible and the reasons of people who instead want to preserve an efficient cooperative scheme. Therefore, the fact that many social structures are designed for people without disability does not lead automatically to claim that all of these social structures are unjust.[34] From this perspective, the Equal Opportunities Model certainly recognizes the social matrix of disability, although not necessarily a form of oppression, and the means to counteract disability would be not only the elimination of social barriers (which should be promoted) but also medical interventions aimed at avoiding some forms of disability in people or future people.

2.4.5   *What Definition of Disability for Procreative Responsibility?*

The analysis of the four models proposed here certainly does not provide definitive answers to the debate on the concept of disability, which would deserve to be investigated in more detailed studies and in a separate context. However, some provisional and general considerations can be drawn, which are helpful for our purposes. Neither the Medical Model nor the Social Model can be considered appropriate tools for defining the concept of disability. On the one hand, the Medical Model fails in conceiving disability as mainly, if not only, related to the bearers of the condition. On the other hand, the Social Model tends to consider psychophysical dysfunction as something not problematic, thus neglecting the experience and the relationship between the individual and their own condition and committing to support the validity of a controversial "right to disability". In addition, the Social Model maintains that the only way to combat the harmed condition experienced by people with disability is to break down social barriers, implicitly theorizing a world completely free of such obstacles. However, this does not consider, first, the impracticability of a world without barriers; second, it does not recognize the demands of non-disabled people who, according to Buchanan, are as legitimate as those of people with disability. In the same direction, although with different arguments, the Welfarist Model believes that it is not possible to indicate the breaking down of social barriers as the only morally acceptable way to counter the consequences of disability since the choice of the methods to counter the negative effects of disability depends on a cost-benefit analysis.

In light of these considerations, the use of medical treatments and interventions in order to treat some forms of disability seems to be "rehabilitated" as an effective tool in this context, although it cannot be considered the only possible instrument. When applied to the procreative context, these considerations could, in some cases, legitimize and demand the use of ARTs as tools aimed at solving or preventing the onset of physical or psychological conditions that are believed could cause a disability in the offspring, considering the conditions of social and natural barriers that the child will face in their life. Although in practice – that is, in the process of defining the conditions of disability in a certain context or society – the Welfarist and Equal Opportunities models often coincide, a methodological distinction nevertheless emerges and should not be overlooked: indeed, understanding the concept of well-being as the fundamental normative element to define the concept of disability may be insufficient, as it does not capture the importance of aspects that transcend psychophysical suffering, such as the limitation of opportunities. Thanks to this discussion of the concept of disability and the limited conclusions I have reached, in Chapter 4, I will be able to define more precisely the notion of harm that will guide the discussion on the contents of procreative responsibility.

Notes

1 This story is found in Vincent (2011) and is an adapted version of Kutz (2004), who in turn adapted his version from Hart (1968/2008).
2 This thought experiment is loosely inspired by Tom Clancy's novel *The Sum of All Fears* (1991).
3 Some may argue that also reasonably foreseeable consequences, but outside the agent's intentions, could in some circumstances be considered outside moral responsibility (Reichlin, 2004).
4 Material capacity in relation to external factors, such as the technological and economic possibilities of performing an action, will be discussed in Section 2.2.
5 Note that being moral agents does not necessarily require that capacity for radical self-determination that the philosophical tradition calls free will. In this regard, see, among others, Frankfurt (1988) and Strawson (2015).
6 Note that in this context, the concept of "moral agent" is not superimposable on the concept of an entity endowed with moral status. It is indeed possible to attribute a certain degree of moral consideration to the mentioned categories, without, however, considering them morally responsible for their own actions. For a deeper understanding of the relationship between moral responsibility, agency, and moral status, see Sebo (2017).
7 Such an aspect raises moral questions regarding the ethics of ignorance (D. J. Miller, 2017). Notice that here I am referring to ignorance of non-moral facts, although other issues could also arise in relation to *moral* ignorance, namely, the condition according to which an agent acts or refrains to act on the basis on what they *mistakenly* believe being morally appropriate. For a discussion on this point, see Harman (2022).
8 Note that, up to this, I accept that omissions can be causes of a state of affairs, but this point is controversial. In this context, I am adhering to the common-sense view that people are responsible for the consequences of at least some omissions, especially when the outcomes of the omissions are as predictable as the outcomes of actions. For instance, a parent might be held responsible for not intervening, when they had the opportunity, to prevent their child from falling from an open window on the fourth floor of the house. It seems reasonable to assert that the child's death crucially depends on the parent's omission. From this, I do not want to delve into the extensive debate over whether omissions can *strictly* cause certain consequences or if they can only be considered meta-causes of an event. Here, I understand causality in broader and general terms, limiting to acknowledge a decisive and undeniable link between a deliberate omission and a subsequent state of affairs. For a discussion, see Clarke (2017, 2022), Dowe (2004), MacKie (1974), and McGee (2011).
9 For a more in-depth discussion, see Kohl (2015).
10 Unlike other taxonomies proposed in the literature, I did not develop in depth the concepts of liability responsibility and virtue responsibility. However, it is

worth mentioning that both depend on the notion of outcome responsibility: an agent assumes responsibility for an event, perhaps through paying a fine, precisely due to the result of their negligence; on the contrary, virtue responsibility relies not on the individual outcome, but on the recurrence of commendable and appreciable results. As noted by Fonnesu, the blame, as a product of outcome responsibility, can indeed signify the recognition of an acting subject's personality or character when they commit either morally wrong or right actions (Fonnesu, 2018). As Vincent suggests, virtue responsibility and virtue irresponsibility – the recurrence of blameworthy results – could significantly influence the definition of liability responsibility (Vincent, 2011).

11 In addition to the technological conditions, it is also possible to consider the economic conditions as factors that determine the material capacity of an agent.

12 For a presentation of classic bioethical problems since the institution of the discipline, see Chadwick and Schüklenk (2020).

13 Note that authors such as Buchanan et al. (2000), Daniels (2008), and David Miller (1979), who argue that increased scrutiny defines a redefinition of our moral duties, refer mainly to issues related to the principle of justice. However, I believe that this argument can also be employed with respect to other moral principles, such as beneficence, non-maleficence, and autonomy.

14 For a critical discussion, see Denier (2010).

15 Moral progress – understood as the set of changes in moral beliefs, practices, and social institutions resulting in a morally desirable state of affairs – is a complex concept that cannot be reduced to just what has been said. In fact, technological development is only one factor that can lead to effective moral progress, but not the only one. For a discussion of this topic, see Buchanan and Powell (2018) and Bina (2023).

16 Notice that in this book when I am claiming that technological development can lead to a redefinition of our moral obligations, I am making a normative evaluation, namely, I am stating that often the increase in material capacities of people brings forth moral reasons to act or not in a certain way. However, the relationship between technological development and moral norms can be also understood in descriptive terms. From this perspective, it can be argued that new technologies may lead to a change in the set of values and duties shared by a community, regardless of whether there are justifications for this change. In this vein, the notion of "techno-moral change" has been introduced. For a discussion, see Rueda (2024).

17 The distinction between concept and conception is further developed by Del Bò (2022).

18 As proof of this trend, think, for example, of the Convention on the Rights of the Child promoted by the United Nations in 1989.

19 Consider, for example, the case of Charlie Gard (Savulescu, 2017; Wilkinson & Savulescu, 2018) or the more recent one of Indi Gregory.

20 Dependency rights are a type of rights that cannot be attributed only to children. They can also be attributed to other vulnerable categories, such as humans with severe cognitive disabilities, prisoners, or even some non-human animals.

21 Notice that in this context, the right to reproduction is not understood as an absolute right, but rather as the possibility of having a reproductive system capable of reproduction.

22 In Chapter 6, I will develop the Child's Right to an Open Future argument with reference to its use in the procreative context.

23 This does not mean being against abortion, as will be discussed in Chapter 4.

24 Note that in my previous works, i.e., Battisti, Gasparetto and Picozzi (2019) and Battisti (2020, 2021), I have used these terms without considering the distinction I am proposing here.

25 Even the first theorist of eugenics, Francis Galton, believed that the genetic improvement measures of society should not be coercively imposed by the institutions, but freely accepted by individuals on the basis of voluntary adherence to the eugenic project understood as a civil religion Galton (1896/2019).

26 It can be argued that certain genetic information, due to its uncertainty and difficulty to manage, should not be communicated to procreators. However, this is a regulatory issue, and it is beyond the scope of this work to discuss it, even though I recognize the importance of regulatory frameworks in shaping the material capacity of an agent and, consequently, procreative responsibility. For insights on communicating genetic information after genetic testing, one can refer to the current discussions on both prenatal and neonatal whole genome sequencing. See, for instance, Battisti (forthcoming), Horton and Lucassen (2022), Thomas et al. (2021), and Johnston et al. (2018).

27 The notion of *prima facie* duty was introduced by William David Ross (1930).

28 In this book, I use *prima facie* moral obligations, *prima facie* moral duties, and moral reasons interchangeably.

29 It is possible to trace this disagreement in the debate not only regarding ARTs but also regarding treatments that could treat deafness after the birth of the child. An example is the cochlear implant, a technology that attempts to "cure" deafness by bypassing the external ear through electrical stimulation of the auditory nerve. To be effective, this treatment must be practiced before the child is fully developed, and this fact raises the question of what the parent should do in these cases. Some activists have called this practice "a cultural genocide". For a philosophical contribution in line with the refusal of this treatment in order to defend the deaf culture, see Sparrow (2005).

30 I will further discuss this case in Chapters 6 and 7.

31 In a similar vein, Camporesi argues that deafness is always an impairment but not a disability (Camporesi, 2010).

32 In this context, some might reply that if P is deaf and the group of which P is a part is a deaf community, P cannot be said to have a disability. In this case, however, the term "group" is understood in broader terms of which deafness community is a sub-group.

33 Buchanan points out that dominant cooperative frameworks (for entire societies) have never been "chosen" in a narrow sense. Rather, they emerged from the cumulative effects of interactions between generations of individuals, rather than from a master plan or collective deliberation. However, in some circumstances, it is possible to exercise a certain degree of choice over some important elements of the schema (Buchanan, 1996).

34 A similar argument is mentioned also by Savulescu and Kahane (2011).

References

Anderson, J. A., Meyn, M. S., Shuman, C., Zlotnik Shaul, R., Mantella, L. E., Szego, M. J., Bowdin, S., Monfared, N., & Hayeems, R. Z. (2017). Parents perspectives on whole genome sequencing for their children: Qualified enthusiasm? *Journal of Medical Ethics*, *43*(8), 535–539.

Anomaly, J. (2014). Public goods and procreation. *Monash Bioethics Review*, 32(3–4), 172–188.

Anomaly, J. (2018). Defending eugenics. *Monash Bioethics Review*. https://doi.org/10.1007/s40592-018-0081-2

Archard, D. (2014). *Children* (3rd ed.). Routledge.

Battisti, D. (2019). Genome editing: Slipping down toward Eugenics? *Medicina Historica*, 3(3), 206–218.

Battisti, D. (2020). Genetic enhancement and the child's right to an open future. *Phenomenology and Mind*, 19, 212.

Battisti, D. (2021). Affecting future individuals: Why and when germline genome editing entails a greater moral obligation towards progeny. *Bioethics*, 35(5), 487–495.

Battisti, D. (forthcoming). Sequenziamento genomico neonatale: quali interessi considerare nella definizione del pannello di geni? *Notizie di Politeia*.

Battisti, D., Gasparetto, A., & Picozzi, M. (2019). Can attitudes toward genome editing better inform cognitive enhancement policy? *AJOB Neuroscience*, 10(1), 59–61.

Bayertz, K. (2003). Human nature: How normative might it be? *The Journal of Medicine and Philosophy*, 28(2), 131–150.

Bennett, R. (2009). The fallacy of the Principle of Procreative Beneficence. *Bioethics*, 23(5), 265–273.

Benston, S. (2016). CRISPR, a crossroads in genetic intervention: Pitting the right to health against the right to disability. *Laws*, 5(1), 5.

Bergnéhr, D. (2009). Social influence and the timing of parenthood. *Interpersona: An International Journal of Personal Relationships*, 3(suppl), 61–83.

Bester, J. C. (2019). The best interest standard and children: Clarifying a concept and responding to its critics. *Journal of Medical Ethics*, 45(2), 117–124.

Bina, F. (2023). *Agency in progress: The ethics, evolution, and psychology of moral change*. Università Vita-Salute San Raffaele. https://iris.unisr.it/handle/20.500.11768/141776

Boorse, C. (1982). On the distinction between disease and illness. In M. Cohen (Ed.), *Medicine and moral philosophy* (pp. 3–22). Princeton University Press.

Bridgeman, J. (2007). *Parental responsibility, young children and healthcare law*. Cambridge University Press.

Brock, D. W. (2005). Shaping future children: Parental rights and societal interests. *The Journal of Political Philosophy*, 13(4), 377–398.

Buchanan, A. (1996). Choosing who will be disabled: Genetic intervention and the morality of inclusion. *Social Philosophy & Policy*, 13(2), 18–46.

Buchanan, A., Brock, D. W., Daniels, N., & Wikler, D. (2000). *From chance to choice*. Cambridge University Press.

Buchanan, A., & Powell, R. (2018). *The evolution of moral progress*. Oxford University Press.

Buller, T., & Bauer, S. (2011). Balancing procreative autonomy and parental responsibility. *Cambridge Quarterly of Healthcare Ethics: CQ: The International Journal of Healthcare Ethics Committees*, 20(2), 268–276.

Cafaro, P. (2012). Climate ethics and population policy. *Wiley Interdisciplinary Reviews. Climate Change*, *3*(1), 45–61.

Camporesi, S. (2010). Choosing deafness with preimplantation genetic diagnosis: An ethical way to carry on a cultural bloodline? *Cambridge Quarterly of Healthcare Ethics: CQ: The International Journal of Healthcare Ethics Committees*, *19*(1), 86–96.

Cane, P. (2003). *Responsibility in law and morality* (2005th ed.). Hart Publishing.

Caruso, G. D. (2018). Consciousness, free will, and moral responsibility.In R. J. Gennaro (Ed.), *The Routledge handbook of consciousness* (pp. 78–91). Routledge.

Cavaliere, G. (2018). Looking into the shadow: The eugenics argument in debates on reproductive technologies and practices. *Monash Bioethics Review*, *36*(1–4), 1–22.

Cavaliere, G. (2020). The problem with reproductive freedom. Procreation beyond procreators' interests. *Medicine, Health Care, and Philosophy*, *23*(1), 131–140.

Chadwick, R. F., & Schüklenk, U. (2020). *This is bioethics*. John Wiley & Sons.

Clarke, R. (2017). *Omissions*. Oxford University Press.

Clarke, R. (2022). Responsibility for acts and omissions. In D. K. Nelkin, & D. Pereboom (Eds.), *The Oxford Handbook of moral responsibility* (pp. 91-C5. P136). Oxford University Press.

Crow, L. (1992). *Renewing the social model of disability*. 5–9 French.

Cutas, D., & Hens, K. (2015). Preserving children's fertility: Two tales about children's right to an open future and the margins of parental obligations. *Medicine, Health Care, and Philosophy*, *18*(2), 253–260.

Dammeyer, J., & Chapman, M. (2018). A national survey on violence and discrimination among people with disabilities. *BMC Public Health*, *18*(1). https://doi.org/10.1186/s12889-018-5277-0

Daniels, N. (2008). *Just health: Meeting health needs fairly*. Cambridge University Press.

Das Gupta, M. (2014). Population, poverty, and climate change. *The World Bank Research Observer*, *29*(1), 83–108.

Davis, D. S. (1997). Genetic dilemmas and the child's right to an open future. *The Hastings Center Report*, *27*(2), 7–15.

Davis, D. S. (2010). *Genetic dilemmas* (2nd ed.). Oxford University Press.

DeGrazia, D. (2016). *Procreative responsibility in view of what parents owe their children* (L. Francis, Ed.). Oxford University Press.

Del Bò, C. (2004). Le questioni di giustizia di fronte alla rivoluzione genetica. *Rivista Di Filosofia*, *95*(1), 141–150.

Del Bò, C. (2022). *La Giustizia. Un'introduzione filosofica*. Carocci.

Denier, Y. (2010). From brute luck to option luck? On genetics, justice, and moral responsibility in reproduction. *The Journal of Medicine and Philosophy*, *35*(2), 101–129.

Dennett, D. C. (2003). *Freedom evolves*. Allen Lane.

Diamond, D. J., & Diamond, M. O. (2017). Parenthood after reproductive loss: How psychotherapy can help with postpartum adjustment and parent–infant attachment. *Psychotherapy (Chicago, IL)*, *54*(4), 373–379.

Donckier, V., Lucidi, V., Gustot, T., & Moreno, C. (2014). Ethical considerations regarding early liver transplantation in patients with severe alcoholic hepatitis not responding to medical therapy. *Journal of Hepatology, 60*(4), 866–871.

Dowe, P. (2004). Causes are physically connected to their effects: Why preventers and omissions are not causes. In C. Hitchcock (Ed.), *Contemporary debates in philosophy of science* (pp. 189–196). Blackwell.

Duff, R. A. (2007). *Answering for crime: Responsibility and liability in the criminal law*. Bloomsbury Publishing.

Farrelly, C. (2002). Genes and social justice: A Rawlsian reply to Moore. *Bioethics, 16*(1), 72–83.

Feinberg, J. (1980). The child's right to an open future. In W. Aiken & H. Lafollette (Eds.), *Whose child?* (pp. 124–153). Rowman & Littlefield.

Fischer, J. M., & Ravizza, M. (1998). *Cambridge studies in philosophy and law: Responsibility and control: A theory of moral responsibility*. Cambridge University Press.

Flatau, L., Reitt, M., Duttge, G., Lenk, C., Zoll, B., Poser, W., Weber, A., Heilbronner, U., Rietschel, M., Strohmaier, J., Kesberg, R., Nagel, J., & Schulze, T. G. (2018). Genomic information and a person's right not to know: A closer look at variations in hypothetical informational preferences in a German sample. *PloS One, 13*(6), e0198249.

Fonnesu, L. (2018). La responsabilità tra teoria e storia. Una proposta. In F. Miano (Ed.), *Etica e responsabilità* (pp. 45–59). Orthotes.

Frankfurt, H. G. (1988). What we are morally responsible for. In H. G. Frankfurt, *The importance of what we care about* (pp. 95–103). Cambridge University Press.

Galton, F. (2019). *Hereditary genius*. Blurb.

Gheaus, A. (2012). The right to parent one's biological baby. *The Journal of Political Philosophy, 20*(4), 432–455.

Harman, E. (2022). Ethics is hard! What follows? On moral ignorance and blame. In D. K. Nelkin, & D. Pereboom, (Eds.), *The Oxford Handbook of moral responsibility* (pp. 327-C16.N35). Oxford University Press.

Harris, J. (2001). One principle and three fallacies of disability studies. *Journal of Medical Ethics, 27*(6), 383–387.

Hart, H. L. A. (2008). *Punishment and responsibility* (2nd ed.). Oxford University Press. (Original work published 1968)

Hart, S. N. (1991). From property to person status: Historical perspective on children's rights. *The American Psychologist, 46*(1), 53–59.

Hasler, F. (1993). Developments in the disabled people's movement. In J. Swain, S. French, C. Barnes, & C. Thomas (Eds.), *Disabling barriers, enabling environments*. Sage.

Häyry, M. (2023). Procreative generosity: Why we should not have children. *Philosophies, 8*(5), 96. https://www.mdpi.com/2409-9287/8/5/96

Hens, K., Cutas, D., & Horstkötter, D. (2017). Parental responsibility: A moving target. In K. Hens, D. Cutas, & D. Horstkötter (Eds.), *Parental responsibility in the context of neuroscience and genetics* (pp. 1–12). Springer International Publishing.

Hickey, C., Rieder, T. N., & Earl, J. (2016). Population engineering and the fight against climate change. *Social Theory and Practice, 42*(4), 845–870.

Hofmann, B. (2017). 'You are inferior!' Revisiting the expressivist argument. *Bioethics, 31*(7), 505–514.

Holm, S. (2008). Parental responsibility and obesity in children. *Public Health Ethics, 1*(1), 21–29.

Horton, R., & Lucassen, A. (2022). Ethical issues raised by new genomic technologies: The case study of newborn genome screening. *Cambridge Prisms: Precision Medicine*, 1–16.

Johnston, J. (2019). "good parents" can promote their own and their children's flourishing. In E. Parens, & J. Johnston (Eds.), *Human flourishing in an age of gene editing* (pp. 112–125). Oxford University Press.

Johnston, J., Lantos, J. D., Goldenberg, A., Chen, F., Parens, E., Koenig, B. A., & members of the NSIGHT Ethics and Policy Advisory Board. (2018). Sequencing newborns: A call for nuanced use of genomic technologies. *The Hastings Center Report, 48*(Suppl 2), S2–S6.

Kant, I. (1929). *Critique of pure reason* (N. K. Smith, Trans.). Mcmillan and Co. (Original work published 1781)

Kohl, M. (2015). Kant and 'ought implies can.' *The Philosophical Quarterly, 65*(261), 690–710.

Kutz, C. (2004). *Chapter 14: Responsibility* (J. Coleman & S. Shapiro, Eds.; pp. 548–587). Oxford University Press.

Loi, M. (2010). Una teoria della giustizia, geneticamente modificata. *Philosophy and Public Issues – Filosofia E Questioni Pubbliche, 14*(1), 161–168.

MacKie, J. L. (1974). *Cement of the universe*. Oxford University Press.

Magni, S. F. (2019). *L'etica tra genetica e neuroscienze. Libero arbitrio, responsabilità, generazione*. Carocci.

McGee, A. J. (2011). Omissions, causation, and responsibility. *Journal of Bioethical Inquiry, 8*(4), 351–361.

Miller, D. (1979). *Social justice*. Oxford University Press.

Miller, D. (2001). Distributing responsibilities. *The Journal of Political Philosophy, 9*(4), 453–471.

Miller, D. J. (2017). "Reasonable Foreseeability and Blameless Ignorance." *Philosophical Studies, 174*(6), 1561–1581.

Mills, C. (2011). *Futures of Reproduction: Bioethics and biopolitics*. Springer Netherlands.

Mitchell, A. M., & Christian, L. M. (2017). Financial strain and birth weight: The mediating role of psychological distress. *Archives of Women's Mental Health, 20*(1), 201–208.

Mitchell, D., & Snyder, S. (2003). The Eugenic Atlantic: Race, disability, and the making of an international Eugenic science, 1800–1945. *Disability & Society, 18*(7), 843–864.

Mori, M. (2020). Il controllo della riproduzione umana come ingresso in una nuova civiltà caratterizzata dalla fertilità come "optional" e da diverse modalità di nascita. *Bioetica Rivista Interdisciplinare, 2–3*, 365–378.

Moss, A. H., & Siegler, M. (1991). Should alcoholics compete equally for liver transplantation? *JAMA: The Journal of the American Medical Association, 265*(10), 1295–1298.

Nelkin, D. K., & Pereboom, D. (Eds.). (2022). *The Oxford handbook of moral responsibility*. Oxford University Press.

Overall, C. (2012). *Why have children?* MIT Press.

Parens, E., & Asch, A. (2003). Disability rights critique of prenatal genetic testing: Reflections and recommendations. *Mental Retardation and Developmental Disabilities Research Reviews, 9*(1), 40–47.

Pinchbeck, I., & Hewitt, M. (1973). *Children in English society volume II*. University of Toronto Press.

Rawls, J. (2009). *A theory of justice* (2nd ed.). Belknap Press.

Reichlin, M. (2004). Il concetto di responsabilità in Bioetica. *Teoria, 1*, 85–103.

Robertson, J. A. (1994). *Children of choice: Freedom and the new reproductive technologies*. Princeton University Press.

Ross, A. (1992). *On guilt responsibility & punishment*. University of California Press.

Ross, W. D. (1930). *The Right and the Good*. Oxford University Press.

Rothman J. C (2010). The challenge of disability and access: reconceptualizing the role of the medical model. *Journal of Social Work in Disability & Rehabilitation. 9*(2), 194–222

Rothman, J. C. (2018). *Social work practice across disability*. Routledge.

Rueda J. (2024). *Disrupting humanity? Anticipatory ethics for genetic enhancement technologies*. University of Granada.

Savulescu, J. (2017). Is it in Charlie Gard's best interest to die? *Lancet, 389*(10082), 1868–1869.

Savulescu, J., & Kahane, G. (2009a). The welfarist account of disability. In K. Brownlee & A. Cureton (Eds.), *Disability and disadvantage* (pp. 14–53). Oxford University Press.

Savulescu, J., & Kahane, G. (2009b). The moral obligation to create children with the best chance of the best life. *Bioethics, 23*(5), 274–290.

Savulescu, J., & Kahane, G. (2011). Disability: A welfarist approach. *Clinical Ethics, 6*(1), 45–51.

Sebo, J. (2017). Agency and moral status. *Journal of Moral Philosophy, 14*(1), 1–22.

Senderovich, H. (2016). How can we balance ethics and law when treating smokers? *Rambam Maimonides Medical Journal, 7*(2), e0011.

Shakespeare, T. (2014). *Disability rights and wrongs revisited* (2nd ed.). Routledge.

Shakespeare, T. (2017). The social model of disability. In L. J. Davis (Ed.), *The disability studies reader* (pp. 195–203). Routledge.

Sparrow, R. (2005). Defending deaf culture: The case of Cochlear implants. *Journal of Political Philosophy, 13*(2), 1467–9760.

Strawson, P. F. (2015). *Freedom and resentment and other essays*. Routledge.

Swierstra, T., & Waelbers, K. (2012). Designing a good life: A matrix for the technological mediation of morality. *Science and Engineering Ethics, 18*(1), 157–172.

Thomas, J., Harraway, J., & Kirchhoffer, D. (2021). Non-invasive prenatal testing: Clinical utility and ethical concerns about recent advances. *The Medical Journal of Australia, 214*(4), 168–170.e1.

UK Law Commission. (1982). *Family law: Illegitimacy, Law Com. No. 118.* Her Majesty's Stationery Office.

Union of the Physically Impaired Against Segregation. (1976). *Fundamental principles of disability.* https://disability-studies.leeds.ac.uk/wp-content/uploads/sites/40/library/UPIAS-fundamental-principles.pdf

van de Poel, I. (2011). The relation between forward-looking and backward-looking responsibility. In N. Vincent, I. van de Poel & J. van den Hoven (Eds.), *Moral responsibility* (pp. 37–52). Springer Netherlands.

Vance, C. (2024). Procreation is Immoral on Environmental Grounds. *The Journal of Ethics, 28*(1), 101–124.

Vincent, N. A. (2011). A structured taxonomy of responsibility concepts. In *Moral responsibility* (pp. 15–35). Springer Netherlands.

Vincent, N. A., & Jane, E. A. (2019). Parental responsibility and gene editing. In *Human flourishing in an age of gene editing* (pp. 126–140). Oxford University Press.

Waelbers, K. (2011). *Doing good with technologies.* Springer.

Wasserman, D. T. (2005). The nonidentity problem, disability, and the role morality of prospective parents. *Ethics, 116*(1), 132–152.

Wendell, S. (1996). *The rejected body. Feminist philosophical reflections on disability.* Routledge.

Wikler, D. (1999). Can we learn from eugenics? *Journal of Medical Ethics, 25*(2), 183–194.

Wilkinson, D., & Savulescu, J. (2018). Hard lessons: Learning from the Charlie Gard case. *Journal of Medical Ethics, 44*(7), 438–442.

Wise, P. H. (2012). Emerging technologies and their impact on disability. *The Future of Children, 22*(1), 169–191.

3 Procreative Beneficence, the Non-Identity Problem, and Impersonal Harm

In previous chapters, I introduced the concept of procreative responsibility, which was defined as the set of *prima facie* moral duties faced by those who are about to generate a new child. As previously noted, there are several procreative responsibility models or principles: the most debated in bioethical discussions is likely the Principle of Procreative Beneficence (PPB) proposed by Julian Savulescu and also defended by others.[1] This chapter will explore this model, aiming to offer convincing reasons to consider it inappropriate for guiding procreative choices. The challenges of PPB presented here will be twofold: critiques that address PPB on its own terms and those that scrutinize its practical normative implications when it comes to balancing various moral reasons inherent in procreation. In other words, PPB may be criticized from both an *internal* perspective and an *external* perspective. While bioethical debates have primarily focused on internal critiques, in this chapter, I also address the external ones, arguing that they represent the most problematic aspects of PPB.

I will begin by providing an accurate formulation of PPB and subsequently examine its implicit assumptions and theoretical premises. This approach is designed to assist readers in analyzing the various models of procreative responsibility discussed herein, enabling them to understand not only the practical implications but also the underlying theories that are essential for grasping various conceptual distinctions.

This chapter is structured as follows: in Section 3.1, I will present PPB by analyzing some of its features. This model, I will argue, is comparative, maximizing, and *prima facie*. After addressing several critiques that consider the model *per se*, I argue that the PPB is an impersonal principle. To unpack this aspect, it will be crucial to explain the Non-Identity Problem introduced by Derek Parfit (1984), which highlights how different moral intuitions in procreative scenarios often contradict each other. In Section 3.2, after introducing this problem, I will discuss several strategies aimed at solving it, pointing out their limitations. I will then discuss one of the most acknowledged strategies in the debate, the maximizing impersonal

DOI: 10.4324/9781032654683-4

strategy, scrutinizing its critical implications, including the well-known Repugnant Conclusion. Given this context, in Section 3.3, I will address the PPB as an impersonal principle, primarily focusing on challenges that arise from the relationship between impersonal reasons and the concept of person-affecting harm in procreative choices.

3.1   The Principle of Procreative Beneficence

According to the most often quoted formulation of the PPB:

> If couples (or single reproducers) have decided to have a child, and selection is possible, then they have a significant moral reason to select the child, of the possible children they could have, whose life can be expected, in light of the relevant available information, to go best or at least not worse than any of the others.
>
> (Savulescu & Kahane, 2009, p. 274)

By "selection", authors typically refer to the use of Preimplantation Genetic Diagnosis (PGD), which can only be undertaken after undergoing *In Vitro* Fertilization (IVF). Proponents of this principle believe there is a moral duty to resort to such practices to select an embryo with(out) certain characteristics. This model does not merely require prospective parents not to transfer embryos with pathological traits during the selection process. As previously mentioned in Chapter 1, in the future, PGD could provide information not only related to monogenic or polygenic diseases but also about non-pathological traits, like intelligence and behavioral traits.[2] According to Savulescu, even this information should be used to make a procreative choice. He imagines a future scenario where it is possible to select embryos based on any genetic trait. In light of this possibility, PPB requires that reproducers maximize the quality of life or well-being of the offspring, promoting a moral duty to select the best or, as more recently defined, the most advantaged possible child. The definition of "the most advantaged child" is not limited to an embryo free from foreseeable genetic diseases, but the distinguishing genetic traits could also include those that might ensure the highest possible well-being for the future individual, such as certain physical or cognitive characteristics.

From this perspective, the advancement of Assisted Reproductive Technologies (ARTs) would significantly expand procreative responsibility. According to Savulescu, there exists a significant moral reason to undergo IVF and, therefore, PGD to select an embryo with an expected higher quality of life than other produced embryos. Moreover, with the introduction of *In Vitro* Gametogenesis (IVG), prospective parents would have a significant moral reason to produce a large-scale number of embryos to have more chance of finding embryos with desired traits. Choosing specific genetic traits from 10 embryos after traditional IVG plus PGD might yield inferior results compared to selecting from 1,000 embryos made possible by IVG (Bourne et al., 2012).

According to its proponents, PPB is neutral concerning the definition of a better life or a good life and does not rely on a specific or controversial conception of well-being. Instead, it requires us to apply the same concepts we already employ in everyday situations to our procreative decisions.

At first glance, it seems the responsibility envisioned by PPB is primarily understood as a parental duty to maximize the well-being of the future individual. According to this interpretation, PPB should be considered a procreative-parental responsibility model and not a mere reproductive responsibility model since it would encompass the obligations of the parent-to-be toward their future child. However, in Subsection 3.3.1, I will provide reasons to consider PPB merely as a reproductive responsibility model.

Intuitively, the idea of having to choose the child with the "best" traits may seem a radical and morally problematic request, as it contrasts with the moral duty to accept the future child as a gift of Nature or God (Sandel, 2009). However, Savulescu and Guy Kahane – co-authors of the most recent and significant papers on PPB (2009, 2016) – argue that PPB is clearly aligned with commonsense morality and our intuitions regarding the concept of parental responsibility. Many believe that parents have moral reasons to be concerned about the potential well-being of their future child. If this premise is accepted, parents should also aim to select the more advantaged child rather than leaving this selective choice to chance or nature. Just as many find it morally problematic not to consider one's personal, financial, and health situation when deciding when to have a child, it would be equally controversial not to use new reproductive tools to select an individual with the highest expected well-being.

3.1.1 Characteristics of the Principle of Procreative Beneficence

Three features of PPB are worth clarifying at the outset. First, it does not require parents to create the perfect child or a child more advantaged than other existing children. This would expose it to criticism, according to which PPB would require parents to refrain from having a child if this child had a less advantaged existence or lesser well-being than other existing children. On the contrary, PPB prescribes selecting the future child – among those possible for the parents given their genetic heritage – whose life one can expect to contain the greatest possible well-being. For this reason, PPB is defined as a *comparative* model.

Second, PPB is a *maximizing* principle since it claims that the morally appropriate selective choice is the one that maximizes the well-being of the future individual. However, it would be naive not to recognize that it is extremely unlikely that a parent would know which child will enjoy greater well-being or have the best life; in fact, individuals born with extraordinary gifts and talents can waste them, while those born with great difficulties can overcome enormous obstacles. For this reason, the maximization required by PPB aims not at final well-being but at *expected* well-being, based on the assumption that someone who has, for example, excellent health and marked intelligence can more easily experience a higher quality of life.

Third, in line with what I argued in the previous chapter, PPB implies no absolute moral duty but *prima facie* ones. It does not prescribe what would always be morally right to do, but only what prospective parents have a significant moral reason to do. However, there are other morally relevant reasons to consider in procreative choices, such as the well-being of prospective parents or other people. According to Savulescu and Kahane, morality consists of choosing to do what we have the most reasons to do (Savulescu & Kahane, 2009). In the procreative context, this means balancing the reasons arising from PPB and others in contrast to the former and assessing, before making a choice, which reasons are the most compelling.

It is worth noting that Savulescu, in his early works, does not explicitly distinguish between moral and non-moral reasons (Savulescu, 2001); this is rather controversial because it confuses the moral dimension with the prudential one without providing a reason to justify this overlap. This overlap is also problematic because it exposes Savulescu's conception of morality to the interpretation that there is a moral obligation to act in light of a balance of *all* reasons, but this seems absurd. Andrew Hotke offers an example where a person has more reasons to have breakfast than to skip it. If morality requires them to act considering all reasons, moral and non-moral, then it would be morally wrong for them to skip breakfast (Hotke, 2014). A more appropriate interpretation, especially in light of more recent works in which PPB has been defended, argues that the reasons to balance should be moral in nature.

Note also that the *prima facie* moral obligation emerging from PPB does not translate into a legal sanction. This makes the principle compatible with respect for procreative autonomy and the right to make choices that could foreseeably result in the generation of a child with suboptimal expected well-being. In this context, the validity of PPB is consistent with a legal system that allows, for example, deaf people to have a deaf child, as in the already mentioned case of Sharon Duchesneau and Candy McCullough, a choice defended by Savulescu himself (2002). But this does not mean that some lawful choices made by parents are not, according to the proponents of PPB, "still profoundly wrong" (Savulescu & Kahane, 2009, p. 279).

Nevertheless, we should notice that selecting a child with deafness may be compatible with PPB in certain, quite limited and unlikely, circumstances: it may be permissible when prospective parents must choose between embryos that are all predisposed to deafness or when selecting for deafness is a way to choose the most advantaged child due to the context in which the future child will grow up. This is because some may argue that a connection to community and family is only possible through shared deafness.[3]

Understanding PPB as *prima facie* or *pro tanto* moral obligation allows us, finally, to understand why the supporters of this principle focus more on some reproductive selective practices and not on others. The focus is primarily on PGD; however, elective abortion can also be conceived as a selective practice. Consider the following example:

> Geneva and Blake passionately want to have a child. The pregnancy progresses normally, but in the second month, after undergoing Non-Invasive Prenatal Testing, they discover that the fetus has a chromosomal disorder, even though there is no risk of miscarriage. Doctors assured them that if they decided to abort, they would have a good chance of conceiving a new child not affected by such a disorder.[4]

Although, in this case, the possible future children are not all already present at the time of choice – unlike the case where the reproducer must choose between two or more embryos – I argue that we are still faced with a form of selection. Therefore, I argue that PPB supporters are committed to arguing that the prescriptions of the principle should also be considered in these circumstances. Hence, according to PPB, there would be significant moral reasons in favor of Geneva and Blake choosing to abort in order to produce the most advantaged child possible. Given the characteristics and statement of the principle, considering the validity of PPB only in the case of PGD and not in elective abortion would be an irremediably *ad hoc* move.

A valid alternative argument to support the applicability of PPB only to PGD and not to abortion is to consider the fetus, unlike the early embryo, already a person. In this context, while *in vitro* selective practice would not raise moral issues related to the dignity of the embryo, abortion would be considered morally problematic. Nevertheless, this does not seem to be the path Savulescu and colleagues want to take.

So why do supporters of PPB mainly refer to PGD rather than extending this reasoning to elective abortion? The reason seems to be that Savulescu and colleagues consider abortion potentially more emotionally and physically burdensome for the pregnant person and the couple compared to PGD; therefore, although the PPB prescriptions continue to apply in this context, the significant reasons in contrast to the implementation of such a principle are particularly compelling (Savulescu, 2001).

As will be seen later, Savulescu and Kahane (2016) recognize that even in the context of PGD, the burdens for the couple and, especially, the psycho-physical ones for the pregnant person can play a decisive role in procreative choices. The requirements of PPB could also be "defused" not only by the physical and emotional burdens that the pregnant person might experience during an abortion but also by the particular moral perspective concerning the fetus that the pregnant person and the couple find convincing. As the same supporters of the model under examination state: "The scope of the principle will depend on our stand on moral questions about [...], IVF, abortion, or the moral status of embryos" (Savulescu & Kahane, 2016, p. 278). Subsection 3.3.3 will discuss the problematic relationship between the moral reasons emerging from PPB and the other issues at stake in selective procreative choice.

According to the authors, considering that PPB generates *prima facie* moral duty allows it to be considered alongside other reasons for beneficence, such as caring for the well-being of future generations, which must be weighed against other moral considerations. This especially helps us to understand that this principle cannot be considered unconditional. It should be noted, moreover, that PPB was not explicitly considered a *prima facie* principle in its initial formulations. This led some bioethicists to criticize PPB as an "absolute" moral duty (de Melo-Martin, 2004). However, especially in light of the already discussed issue regarding abortion, I believe that understanding the PPB prescriptions as *pro tanto* moral reasons is an element that has been present, at least implicitly, in all formulations of the principle.

3.1.2   *Internal Criticisms of the Principle of Procreative Beneficence*

PPB has been widely criticized. Such criticisms can be of two types: internal and external. In this subsection, I will discuss the internal criticisms, which consider PPB in itself, that is, the challenges of the idea that a prospective parent has a significant moral reason to select the best possible child. Without claiming to provide an exhaustive discussion, I will report the most important criticisms, sometimes accompanied by some rebuttals by Savulescu and Kahane that appear particularly convincing.

3.1.2.1   *The Eugenic Criticism*

According to Robert Sparrow (2007) and Rebecca Bennett (2009), PPB would imply coercion or, at least, would implicitly invite the use of coercive tools for parents to select the best possible child. Despite the claims of its proponents that PPB entails no coercion and is compatible with a libertarian conception of reproductive choices, some have argued that PPB is, in fact, coercive. Advocating for a moral duty to have the most advantaged child puts a lot of pressure on individuals to pursue this goal (Bennett, 2009). Sparrow goes further, arguing that Savulescu should be committed to the view that there are substantial *prima facie* reasons for the State to enforce the obligation implied by PPB. When a moral obligation such as that generated by PPB is openly disregarded, it could mark the start of a rationale suggesting that State intervention may be necessary to correct this situation. The case for such intervention gains momentum with the increase of significance of the obligation for a specific society (Sparrow, 2007). Furthermore, once reproductive Genome Editing (rGE) becomes possible and available, PPB would imply the moral imperative not only to select the best child among those available but also to resort to genetic enhancement through engineering (Anomaly & Johnson, 2023; Gantsho, 2022; Sparrow, 2011; Veit, 2018).[5]

The criticism of a slippery slope toward new coercive eugenics would need to be supported by more solid empirical arguments to be effective against PPB. The emphasis contemporary society puts on the private nature of human reproduction, the great importance placed on procreative freedom by society in recent decades, and the condition of factual pluralism on the different conceptions of good and well-being observable within our society cast doubt on the validity of this criticism in Western societies.[6] It should also be clarified that Savulescu and Kahane's intention is to discuss the emerging moral obligations of future parents, not what the State or other institutions should try to impose or prevent (Savulescu & Kahane, 2016). Nevertheless, it is reasonable to argue that PPB logically implies a certain moral obligation to resort to genetic enhancement, where possible, even if PPB's supporters might not consider this aspect a real criticism.[7]

3.1.2.2 *The Expressivist Objection*

Some argue that PPB would be open to the already discussed expressivist objection, according to which people with disabilities would be conferred a lower value and would be discriminated against. Even granting that the potential use of ARTs to select an individual based on prospective parents' preferences does not necessarily discriminate against people with disabilities (Buchanan, 1996), it should be acknowledged that the imposition of a moral obligation to select the best possible individual would create a hierarchy between better lives and suboptimal lives. Therefore, some may argue that these putative moral reasons would discriminate against the community of people with disabilities in a new way compared to the mere possibility of using ARTs to promote the procreative freedom of reproducers. Note that this criticism could be extended beyond PPB to other models of procreative responsibility that impose some constraints on procreators' freedom. It is outside the scope of this work to address the expressivist argument extensively. Here, I just wanted to highlight the greater efficacy of the argument in the context of procreative obligations rather than in the use of ARTs to support reproductive freedom. In the latter scenario, a value judgment is not necessarily involved: prospective parents may avoid having a child with a disability not due to a perceived lower value of people with disabilities but because it does not align with their personal life plans. However, such value judgment could be implied in the context of procreative obligation. That said, the considerations made in Section 2.4 regarding the definition of disability and procreative responsibility offer a valuable starting point for addressing this critical aspect of procreative ethics.

3.1.2.3   *The Internal Normativity Criticism*

Other authors have challenged the model's actual capacity to be normative. According to Ben Saunders, Savulescu fails to show that PPB implies a genuine moral obligation because this model confuses the concept of a *moral reason* with that of a *moral obligation* (Saunders, 2015). According to Savulescu and Kahane, these concepts can be considered synonymous:

> Those who prefer to think of such reasons as generated by moral obligations should also think of reasons of [P]PB as generated by an obligation. Since we do not think that anything turns on this distinction, in what follows we will use moral reason and moral obligation interchangeably.
> (Savulescu & Kahane, 2009, p. 278)

However, many argue that, in certain circumstances, people have moral reasons but no moral obligation to perform a certain action. For example, one may have moral reasons to donate every dollar to counteract global poverty but not a moral duty to act in this way. From this perspective, according to Saunders, PPB would seem to implicitly support the non-existence of supererogatory actions, where a supererogatory action is understood as a "noble" action, not imperative, that cannot be required of everyone. Thus, even admitting that parents have moral reasons to choose the child with the expected best life, there might not exist a moral obligation to act in this direction (Saunders, 2015). Here, moral reason and moral obligation are not used as synonyms: whereas the notions of moral obligation capture what is something that is mandatory, moral reasons refer to what is simply morally good but not imperative. This criticism evokes a general objection to utilitarian positions. The relationship between PPB and the utilitarian perspective will be further clarified in Subsections 3.2.2 and 3.3.2.

3.1.2.4 The Criticism of the Comparative Feature

PPB can also be criticized through an argument that challenges its comparative feature. In fact, Savulescu provides no reason why PPB should only prescribe parents to select the future child – among those possible for the parents given their genetic inheritance – from which the greatest possible well-being can be expected and not the "perfect child". If technological means were available to select or create an individual with better-expected well-being than all others, then, according to this criticism, PPB should prescribe, at least in principle, the selection of such an embryo. Following this observation, Sparrow provocatively notes that PPB would require all parents in a given environment to reproduce using clones of the same embryo, selected to possess the best genome for that particular environment (Sparrow, 2007, 2015). This scenario might be logically plausible but is highly unlikely given how the world works, according to Savulescu and Kahane.

However, even admitting the implausibility of the model's comparative feature, the authors argue that it is compatible with the idea that there is not a single "best" genetic inheritance and, therefore, a precise hierarchical ordering of embryos. In other words, a perfect hierarchy would be absurd (Savulescu & Kahane, 2016). To explain this, Savulescu and Kahane use the following analogy: they ask each of us to imagine the best day of our life. We will likely think of different days, not just one, and it might not be possible to say which was truly the best. However, this does not mean we cannot recognize terrible days or even those that are boring and ordinary. Similarly, while it may be impossible to rank all embryos hierarchically, we can still identify those with greater expected well-being.

3.1.2.5 The Criticism of the Concept of a Better Life

According to Michael Parker, the concept of a better life cannot be reduced to simple elements identifiable through embryo screening (Parker, 2007). If we consider our lives and those of our friends and family, it is extremely hard to precisely indicate in advance, or even in hindsight, what makes or made our life better. Parker believes it is impossible to argue that a life free from troubled interpersonal relationships, free from suffering and loneliness, is overall better than a life where these conditions have occurred to some degree. This suggests that although one can outline traits that might lead to good lives, it is impossible to relate the characteristics of embryos identifiable through PGD with complex concepts such as "a better life" through a ranking of worse or better lives. This means that "the best possible expected life" is impossible to determine.

According to Savulescu, Parker's criticism is not an objection to PPB but to the broader argument that it is possible to assign value to life. Saying life cannot be evaluated means accepting that it is impossible to establish priorities in health, research, social services, and the distribution of limited resources. Even if definite rankings might not be possible, it does not follow that partial "rankings" cannot exist. Even admitting that it might not be possible to say whether A is better than B, it might still be possible to say that A and B are better than C. This is enough to rationally reject C. There will be constellations of traits that will be inferior to others, and this is enough for PPB to be valuable (Savulescu, 2007).

3.1.2.6 The Criticism of the Neutrality of the Definition of Well-Being

There is another problematic aspect related to the concept of well-being underlying the principle. Savulescu and Kahane (2009) claim to embrace a neutral concept of a good life since they are aware that this notion is extremely personal and subjective or tied to some highly debatable ideal of human flourishing. According to Massimo Reichlin, however, because of this choice, PPB ends up reducing the scope of its prescriptions to avoiding diseases burdened by well-defined pathological conditions, something quite different from selecting the most advantaged child possible (Reichlin, 2012). By assuming a certain neutrality about the concept of a good life, PPB would collapse into another model proposed in the literature, the N Principle, supported by Allen Buchanan and colleagues: according to this model, parents would not be morally obligated to select the best possible child, but any child who will not "suffer severe pain, limited opportunities, or a significant loss of happiness or good" (Buchanan et al., 2000, p. 249). On the contrary, according to Reichlin, PPB would work better if it accepted an objective theory of well-being but would expose itself to the criticisms that this theory would bring up. The more the subjectivity of the concept of well-being is emphasized, the more the definition of a better life is deprived of precise meaning, thereby removing the novel, prescriptive perspective suggested by PPB proponents. It should be noted, however, that Savulescu and Kahane have tried to defend a partially objectivist theory, arguing that characteristics and capabilities of people relating to objective goods should be sought and preserved, such as the ability to establish deep personal relationships (Savulescu & Kahane, 2011, 2016; Savulescu et al., 2014).

3.2 The Non-Identity Problem

In addition to the characteristics described in the previous pages, there is another feature of PPB that is central and even more important than the considerations reported so far. Before being a comparative, maximizing, and *prima facie* model, PPB is primarily an "impersonal" one. To understand what "impersonal" means in this context, it is necessary to introduce one of the most paradigmatic philosophical issues of the second half of the 20th century, which is crucial for the definition of procreative responsibility: the Non-Identity Problem.

The Non-Identity Problem was raised, seemingly independently, in the second half of the 1970s by Derek Parfit (1976), Thomas Schwarz (1978), and Robert Adams (1979). However, its most systematic and influential treatment can be traced back to Parfit's book *Reasons and Persons* (1984).

Parfit observes that a choice in the present that affects the lives of future people can be of three kinds: a choice can have effects on the same people (*same people choice*); it can cause one person rather than another to come into existence, namely, affecting the identity of future people (*same number choice*); or it can have effects both on the identity and the number of future people (*different number choice*). The Non-Identity Problem arises when agents' choices determine not only the well-being of future individuals but also their identity.

In discussing the Non-Identity Problem, Parfit understands identity in the numerical sense. Generally, numerical identity is the relationship that an entity has with itself and with nothing else. Numerical identity is distinct from qualitative identity: an object is qualitatively identical to another object when they are exactly alike: one is a replica of the other. However, the two objects cannot be numerically identical; referring to one or the other does not refer to the same object. To better illustrate the difference between the two concepts, Parfit asks us to imagine two white billiard balls: they cannot be said to be numerically identical but can be considered qualitatively identical. However, if we focus on one of the balls and color it red, it is easy to see that it is no longer qualitatively identical to the white ball it once was; however, the white ball at time t1 and the red ball at time t2 share a relationship of numerical identity with each other; that is, they are the same ball (Parfit, 1984, pp. 201–202).

In light of this, Parfit claims that every person has a distinctive necessary property, namely, that of having grown from a specific embryo, which results from the encounter between an oocyte and a sperm cell. Parfit defines this interpretation of identity as the Origin View (Parfit, 1984, p. 352). As in the example of the balls, an individual can be said to be qualitatively different either from their self 10 years ago or from the embryo from which they developed, while still maintaining a relationship of numerical identity with all its versions over time.[8]

Once the concept of identity is defined, we should assess in which cases the agents' choices determine the identity of individuals. To answer this question, consider the following example:

Eddie and Anna want to have a child, but they discover that Anna has rubella. Their doctor informs them that if they were to conceive now, their child would be born deaf and blind. If they chose to wait three months, they would conceive a healthy child. The couple decides to conceive a few days later, giving birth to a child with the aforementioned conditions.[9]

The claim that Eddie and Anna performed a morally wrong action aligns with most people's moral intuitions. Many may think that the couple *harmed* her child by not waiting three months before conceiving. This intuition can also be found in the famous case provided by Parfit, in which a 14-year-old girl decides to have a child (Parfit, 1984). Similar to Anna and Eddie's case, many believe that the girl should wait some time before procreating so as not to give her future child a bad start in life. She should wait, for example, until she has economic, personal, and social stability to ensure her child a better start. However, there is a problem in these two examples, namely, that neither Anna and Eddie's child nor the 14-year-old girl's child seem to have been genuinely disadvantaged by their mothers' choices and, therefore, harmed by them.

One of the most plausible definitions of what it means to "harm someone" states that an act harms a person if they find themselves in a worse situation than they would have been if that act had not been committed.[10] The concept of harm is generally understood as a comparative and counterfactual notion: person P can be said to have been harmed by the occurrence of X when the absence of X would have resulted in a state of affairs in which P would have been better off. Therefore, there is a comparison between at least two possible worlds: (a) P that suffers X and (b) P that does not suffer X. In more general terms, this understanding assesses harm by comparing what happened with what would have happened in a counterfactual situation (Immerman, 2022). There are objections to this account, as well as several versions that attempt to accommodate the objections and disagree about what counterfactual situation or situations are relevant to discussing harm. But this definition still seems to capture what is at stake in the Non-Identity Problem, namely, that to talk about personal harm, we need to have the same person P across the possible counterfactual alternatives that we use to evaluate the occurrence of harm by comparing them (Tomlin, 2022).[11]

In the examples mentioned earlier, such a comparison is not possible because the prospective parents' choices determine not only the condition of their future children but also their identity. In this context, the deaf and blind child could not exist except under those conditions. Action X (deciding to have a deaf and blind child) determines the very identity of the future individual. There is no alternative state of affairs in which the same child, deaf and blind, exists without these characteristics. Therefore, in the analyzed cases, the prospective parents' choices do not seem to have "worsened" the conditions of their children.

At this point, Parfit asks: when we recognize that the mothers did not worsen the conditions of their children, do we change our minds about considering their actions morally wrong? Do we cease to believe that it would have been better if these women had waited to conceive in order to conceive a healthy child or one with a better start? (Parfit, 1984, p. 539). Parfit believes that the conviction that the mothers did something wrong remains, but also recognizes that it is not possible to defend this conviction in the most intuitively compelling way, that is, by arguing that the children were harmed by the prospective parents' choice. So, what is the reason for this morally negative judgment? This question arises because, in different outcomes, numerically different people would be born.[12]

The Non-Identity Problem is not only evident in procreative cases but also manifests in other situations. Parfit provides an example through the case of a Risky Policy. He imagines a community that must decide between two distinct energy policies: Policy A and Policy B. Both policies ensure that the community will survive for at least three centuries. However, Policy A is more high-risk compared to Policy B, even though the former would provide some short-term benefits. Specifically, Policy A involves burying nuclear waste in areas with no risk of earthquakes for the upcoming centuries. However, as this waste will remain radioactive for thousands of years, future risks do exist. That said, if the community chooses Policy A, they will experience a slight increase in their overall well-being and standard of living compared to choosing Policy B.

Eventually, the community decides to adopt Policy A, leading to an environmental catastrophe in the distant future. Due to geological shifts on Earth's surface, an earthquake releases radiation that kills thousands of people. Even though they were killed by this catastrophe, these individuals had led decent lives. Moreover, Parfit assumes that this radiation only affects those born after its release, giving them an incurable disease that will kill them around the age of 40. This disease does not manifest any symptoms before it leads to the death of such people (Parfit, 1984, pp. 371–372). In this scenario as well, it is challenging to argue that the people who died due to radiation were harmed by the community's decision centuries earlier to choose Policy A. After all, if the community had not chosen policy A, those who died around the age of 40 because of radiation would never have existed. The well-being increase provided by Policy A influenced the reproductive choices of the community's citizens. Consequently, the individuals born were numerically different from those who would have existed if the community had chosen Policy B. Yet, this moral conclusion is in stark contrast to the intuitive belief that the community did something profoundly wrong.

The Non-Identity Problem, therefore, poses a challenge because it produces a conclusion that seems to be at odds with commonly held moral beliefs. Specifically, a deeply intuitive moral judgment asserts that an act can be wrong only if it makes things worse for or harms someone (Roberts, 2019). Following the terminology introduced by Parfit, we may call this a *person-affecting intuition*. However, this judgment appears to clash with the conclusion many people arrive at that both the prospective parents from the previous examples and the community made morally wrong choices. The tension between the assumptions or premises of the argument and its conclusion, which conflicts with many people's moral intuitions, gives rise to the Non-Identity Problem. The logical conclusion derived from the mentioned examples – which are referred to as non-identity cases (Johansson, 2019; Višak, 2018; Williams, 2013) – is opposite to what appears to be accepted by common belief, leading to a moral paradox.

3.2.1 Solving the Non-Identity Problem? Some Strategies

To reject what David Boonin (2014) labels the Implausible Conclusion – that is, the conclusion that Anna and Eddie did nothing wrong in conceiving a deaf-blind child – and thereby solve the Non-Identity Problem, various strategies have been proposed. It is beyond the scope of the book to provide a comprehensive discussion of the strategies that have been proposed in the literature.[13] Here, I present some of them before moving on to the discussion of impersonal strategy in Subsection 3.2.2. Such strategies try to demonstrate that in non-identity cases, the resulting child is harmed or wronged by the procreative parents' decisions. For ease of presentation, I will consider only Anna and Eddie's case, even though these arguments can also be applied to the case of the 14-year-old girl and the Risky Policy scenario.

3.2.1.1 Existence and Non-Existence

First, one might argue that accepting this premise would mean endorsing a comparison that is unsustainable. To claim that the child is not disadvantaged by the couple's choice implies a comparison between the situation where the child exists and the situation where the same child does not. However, for many, it is not plausible to compare existence with non-existence. Since such a comparison does not seem feasible, claiming that the child is not disadvantaged simply makes no sense. Even if one accepts that the two situations are incomparable, this alone does not dismiss the Non-Identity Problem. If we assume the incomparability of the two situations, which prevents us from saying the deaf and blind child is not worse off due to the couple's decision, it is also necessary to note that we cannot claim the child is worse off due to the couple's decision; therefore, this strategy does not help in resolving the problem (Boonin, 2008).

3.2.1.2 *The Concept of a Life Not Worth Living*

The second strategy we discuss consists of arguing that, due to her congenital conditions, Anna and Eddie's child has a life so full of suffering that it is not worth living. Although the condition in which Anna and Eddie's child is found is the only one in which this individual could have come into the world, bringing such a person into the world would constitute a morally wrong action. From this perspective, even granting that comparing existence and non-existence is not possible, we may argue that a life overwhelmed by suffering is certainly bad for the child.

Although there is broad consensus among authors that the necessary condition for morally responsible procreation is that the child is reasonably expected to have a life worth living, this does not seem to help much in solving the Non-Identity Problem. The idea of a life not worth living is highly controversial, and it is usually associated with extremely rare illnesses where suffering overwhelmingly surpasses any positive experience (Harris, 1990). In these cases, the child's life is exhaustively predetermined, making it impossible to pursue all current and future goals, whatever they may be (Buller & Bauer, 2011; Steinbock & McClamrock, 1994). This is more evident in cases where someone suffers from profound cognitive and physical disabilities. While it s reasonable to argue that it is hard, if not impossible, to draw a clear, non-arbitrary line between lives worth living and those not, as David DeGrazia highlights, it is also clear enough that some lives are worth living and others are not (DeGrazia, 2016). Setting aside some religious views, such as Christian ones that see every life as worth living, most would agree that lives with disabilities like blindness, deafness, or Down syndrome are undoubtedly worth living, while lives affected by devastating diseases like Lesch–Nyhan syndrome or Tay–Sachs disease are good candidates for the notion of a life not worth living.[14]

Although being deaf and blind entails challenges in relating to others and the environment, it would be controversial to claim that the child is disadvantaged by the couple's choice based on the belief that a life with deaf-blindness is not worth living. Many individuals with these traits are active members of society. According to a 2019 qualitative study investigating the experiences of individuals with this condition, being deaf and blind does not make their lives "unbearable" (Ehn et al., 2019). Thus, claiming that Anna and Eddie's child has a life not worth living does not seem a viable path to justify the intuition that the mother's choice worsened the child's condition.

Instead, it is true that the child's life might become so unbearable that it is considered not worth living, but this is not unique to those with deaf-blindness. Merely by living, all individuals are exposed to traumas, diseases, and psycho-physical sufferings, sometimes independent of initial conditions. Notably, those who request assisted suicide or euthanasia often state that their physical or psychological conditions, typically resulting from severely debilitating diseases with significant impact on their quality of life, have rendered their lives not worth living (Dees et al., 2011). For this reason, in non-identity cases and reproductive scenarios, we speak of conditions that *predictably* make life worthy or not worthy of being lived. Catastrophic diseases such as those presented above could, therefore, make non-existence preferable to existence, contrary to the condition of deaf-blindness, however complex.

In summary, even admitting that some lives are not worth living and that this is a valid reason to consider the generation of such lives morally wrong,[15] this argument does not offer a viable strategy to address the Non-Identity Problem in many cases where procreative choices determine an individual's identity. Instead, this viewpoint might only be valid in rare circumstances and not in most cases where the Non-Identity Problem arises, namely, when the individual generated has a life worth living. When discussing the Non-Identity Problem through various examples, including some already mentioned, Parfit always specifies that the lives of individuals whose existence has been determined by morally scrutinized choices are worth living.

3.2.1.3   *The De Dicto/De Re Distinction*

Another strategy trying to explain that Anna and Eddie's child is wronged by the couple's decision is to argue that the one who is disadvantaged is not the specific individual, but the individual who occupies the position of "child" generated by Anna and Eddie (*same-place holder*), since another individual in different conditions could have been born in their place. This strategy has been defended, among others, by Caspar Hare (2007) and, more recently, by Joona Räsänen (2023), using the distinction between considering the child in a *de re* sense and in a *de dicto* sense. Consider the sentence "Anna and Eddie make their child deaf-blind"; this sentence can be interpreted in two different ways: in the *de re* interpretation, a specific individual is made deaf-blind, instead of being sighted and hearing, by the mother; however, in the *de dicto* interpretation, the couple decides to have a deaf-blind child and thus decides to make "her child", i.e., the one who will hold the place of their child in the world, deaf-blind rather than having a child with different characteristics as "their child". From this perspective, while Anna and Eddie's child is not disadvantaged *de re*, they would be *de dicto*. Therefore, understanding the child in the *de dicto* sense would resolve the Non-Identity Problem. This distinction can be adopted based on two different arguments. The first is based on the claim that the identity of individuals in non-identity cases should not be conceived as the result of the encounter between an oocyte and a sperm cell, as suggested by the Origin View, but in the *de dicto* sense. Although there is some discussion aiming to rehabilitate this interpretation of identity (Williams, 2013; Wolf, 2009), according to Parfit, it seems quite implausible, so much so that it is not worth a thorough refutation:

> This claim meets the objection that each person's life might have been very different. But this claim is also too implausible to be worth discussing. I am the second of my mother's three children. This claim implies absurdly that, if my mother had conceived no child when she in fact conceived me, I would have been my younger sister.
>
> (Parfit, 1984, p. 354)

The second way to understand this distinction is proposed by Caspar Hare, who claims the Non-Identity Problem can be solved by noticing that betterness and worseness can be interpreted in both *de re/de dicto* senses and that the latter one grasps some fundamental aspects of commonsense morality. Focusing solely on harm and benefit toward specific individuals fails to recognize some responsibilities that can be understood in an eminently *de dicto* sense and appear plausible in our moral discourse. Anna and Eddie's case falls in this category. However, to demonstrate this, we need at least an example in which *de dicto* betterness and wrongness are not controversial, and then we need to trace a moral analogy with Anna and Eddie's case. According to Caspar Hare, *de dicto* considerations are morally relevant in cases like the following:

> Tess is a state safety officer, whose job it is to regulate those features of the automobile that protect its occupants in the event of a collision – air bags, crumple zones, and so forth. Noticing that people in her state are not wearing safety belts, she implements some tough new regulations and, a year later, is pleased to discover evidence that they have been effective, that the severity of injuries sustained in automobile accidents has been reduced as a result of people belting up. She gives herself a pat on the back.
>
> (C. Hare, 2007, p. 516)

In this example, Tess' new regulations clearly seem to improve things for people having road accidents. Hare assumes that the regulations affect not only the severity of injuries that occur in accidents but also the identity of those involved in the accident. The new rules might affect the time it takes for each person to start their vehicle, which in turn affects when they reach intersections, red lights, etc. Indeed, due to Tess' regulations, people involved in accidents might not have been involved if the rules had not been implemented. Therefore, according to a *de re* interpretation, Tess did a terrible job: her regulation led some people to have accidents, albeit mild, that without regulation, they would not have had at all.

However, we still think that Tess did an excellent job. According to Caspar Hare, the explanation rests on the plausibility of *de dicto* betterness and wrongness. They are morally relevant when two conditions are met: first, the agent has some role responsibility toward a group of people, as Tess has some responsibilities toward accident victimis; second, the concerns toward the group cannot be expressed in *de re* terms, due to the non-identity circumstances. Caspar Hare argues that these conditions also applie in the case of Anna and Eddie since the couple holds role responsibility, as parents, for their child's health, and Anna and Eddie's case cannot be framed in *de re* terms. Therefore, if Tess' obligation stands, an obligation to wait to procreate for Anna and Eddie also stands.

This argument can be challenged from several perspectives. Boonin, for example, notes that Tess' statement that "my job is to make things *de dicto* better for the victims of the accident" can be interpreted in two ways: (a) Tess made sure that the victims of the accident suffered less harm than would have been suffered by people who would have had car accidents without new regulations; and (b) Tess ensured that the accident victims were the people with a higher level of health after the accident than people who would have had car accidents without new regulation. If Tess' role is (a), then it seems implausible to find any *de dicto* obligation in Anna and Eddie's case, since the couple's duty is simply to minimize the harm suffered by whoever fills the role of their child. The act of procreation, however, does not harm any child, regardless of its characteristics, and therefore no child in *de re* sense among the possible children that the couple could have. If instead (b) is valid, then Anna and Eddie's obligation not to conceive a child for three months could hold, since this means selecting the embryo with a potentially higher level of health. Nevertheless, (b) seems implausible: it would be absurd to claim that Tess's task should be to maximize the future health of accident victims based on their health before the accidents rather than to minimize the accident's severity without considering the drivers' prior health condition (Boonin, 2014).

So, in order to justify an obligation for Anna and Eddie to postpone procreation, a more plausible example in which there is an uncontroversial conclusion based on *de dicto* betterness or worseness is needed. Recently, Räsänen noticed that the Safety Officer's case fails to be on par with Anna and Eddie's case since Tess does not know – and cannot know – the state of health of possible accident victims before they have the accident. It is precisely for this reason that (b) seems rather implausible to us. However, there are plausible cases in which, knowing the level of health expected from our decisions, an obligation similar to (b) may also arise. Räsänen proposes the following example:

Infected Water. Lisa is a water inspector, and her job is to supervise the water distribution to the city. One day, when the safety features of the water supply are temporarily disabled, she finds out that water contains a nasty bacterium, which infects some of the people who drink it and causes them to have severe pain and discomfort. Lisa has two options. She could direct water to Suburbicon, an area of healthy and wealthy people. Call residents of Suburbicon strong. Or she could direct water to Shacktown, an area of the sick and poor. Call residents of Shacktown weak. If Lisa directs water to Suburbicon many but not every resident of Suburbicon get sick and their health is reduced. If Lisa directs water to Shacktown many but not every resident of Shacktown get sick and their health is reduced. If Lisa does nothing, the pressure in the water tank causes the infected water to spread all over the town (because of the disabled safety features) eventually infecting everybody in the Suburbicon and Shacktown! Assuming that the strong possess 100 unit of health and would lose 10 units, and assuming that the weak would lose 5 units of health but they already in less health, say having 60, what should Lisa choose?

(Räsänen, 2023, p. 129)

According to Räsänen, Lisa should direct the water toward the stronger group of people, as it is arguable that Lisa's role is to ensure the eventual victim remains as healthy as possible. If this analogy holds, Anna and Eddie may have reasons to delay procreation. Indeed, since life will always come together with some suffering and harm (Benatar, 2006), there is some reason for Anna and Eddie to delay procreation to put their *de dicto* child in the condition to face suffering stemming from a higher level of health.[16]

Here, I propose a further argument to challenge this approach, arguing that *de dicto/de re* distinction cannot solve the Non-Identity Problem. The two examples provided by Caspar Hare and Räsänen try to persuade us that *de dicto* betterness and wrongness *alone* can provide reasons to argue that Anna should wait to reproduce. They argue that both examples are not explainable in a *de re* sense. But this is a mistake. Indeed, both examples can be understood in *de re* terms more plausibly than in *de dicto* terms, as suggested by the authors. Let us consider the examples one by one: in Tess' case, it seems to me that the primary goal is to avoid serious accidents of people that, after regulation, surely exist, not reducing suffering in whoever will have accidents. Thanks to the new regulation, Tess could indeed prevent specific people from having serious accidents. But these people exist and, accordingly, can experience the fact that Tess spared them from experiencing severe car accidents, being happy for this. It is the existence of such a group of people that essentially prompts Tess to implement new regulations. In other words, Tess' choice assumes that *drivers* can be in two groups, both of which can experience *de re* either suffering or lack of suffering due to happening or not of car accidents. Similarly, when Lisa decides where to direct the water, she considers that another group of people – that will surely exist after Lisa directs – might suffer more than the group with a better level of initial health. This means that the role responsibility of Tess regarding accident victims and that of Lisa in relation to water victims are misunderstood. Tess has a responsibility to *all drivers* to prevent serious accidents, while Lisa has a responsibility to residents of *both* Suburbicon and Shacktown.

This demonstrates that in both cases, we deal with a simple case of allocation of burdens and benefits justifying the suffering caused to *de re* people by Tess and Lisa. In Räsänen's example, this is quite evident: Lisa's choice can be justified by saying the aim was to protect the weaker or the worst off, who otherwise would have had a low health level. The Tess case requires more argumentation: let us assume that in one year in a society made up of 1,000 people where Tess is in charge, there are 500 accidents (a reckless society, though). Tess cannot act on the number of accidents but on where to direct them: toward group A, drivers who will suffer severe accidents, or group B, drivers who will suffer mild consequences after car accidents. If Tess decides to direct the accidents toward A, she can minimize the aggregate suffering in the group of drivers. Moreover, it is plausible that all drivers would accept this measure since at the beginning of the year they still do not know who will end up in group A or group B at the end of the year. All drivers would prudently accept this rule because, in the worst situation where they have an accident, they will find themselves in the best possible position.

Notice, however, that these allocation cases concern benefits and burdens in groups of people that surely will exist after the decision, but this is not the case in Anna and Eddie's story. The latter is more similar to the following: a medical team must decide who to bring into the ICU between two patients, Maximilian and Sergej, who are at risk of death. The decision of practitioners will define whose life they save. Both patients have the same recovery capacity and the same age, but after the ICU treatment, Maximilian is predicted to have a quality of life of 95, whereas Sergej is predicted to have a quality of life of only 65. Excluding social utility considerations that may opt for one or another,[17] it is evident that in this case, practitioners cannot use quality of life as an allocative criterion, except in a utilitarian perspective that Caspar Hare seems to reject. Although both Maximilian and Sergej would prefer a health of 95 over 65, this does not mean that Sergej would rather die than have just 65. If not treated, they both lose all that they possess. Of course, the analogy holds up to a point for obvious reasons – future people do not exist yet, whereas Sergej and Maximilian do – but with this in mind, I claim that while burdens and benefits are allocated over a group of people that will surely exist after the allocative decision, quality-of-life considerations can stand, but when future existence is the object of allocation, this no longer applies. Therefore, the *de dicto* betterness and wrongness fail to explain why Tess and Lisa have moral reasons to act as they did. From this, it does not follow that Anna and Eddie have the same moral reasons to delay reproduction. The Non-Identity Problem is still unresolved.

3.2.2 The Impersonal Strategy

The strategies presented earlier do not seem to lead to a satisfactory resolution of the Non-Identity Problem. For this reason, many philosophers and bioethicists have taken a different path. Their strategy is not to argue that the child has been disadvantaged, harmed, or wronged by the mother's choice. Instead, they claim that some actions or omissions are harmful or wrong even if no individual has been affected by them. From this perspective, the morally correct choice is not only one that specifically benefits, or at least does not harm, someone but also one that makes the world a better place, i.e., a place with a greater amount of aggregate well-being. In this context, we observe that people have moral obligations not only to existing individuals but also to those who could possibly exist. Richard Mervyn Hare refers to the latter as "merely possible persons" (R. M. Hare, 1988), i.e., people who will not exist but could have existed had we chosen differently. Here, harms and benefits are understood not only in comparative terms concerning the same individual but also in comparative terms regarding the lives of merely possible persons. In the moral context, there would thus be harm without a victim, which makes the world a worse place. The specific comparative interpersonal nature required by the concept of impersonal harm prescribes accepting the criteria of substitutability – meaning that actual, possible, and merely possible persons can be replaced by one another – and compensability – meaning that harm done to actual or possible persons can be offset by a benefit given to merely possible persons (Magni, 2019).

For the impersonal strategy to succeed, it must be combined with a plausible normative account of how an act can be wrong even if it does not worsen things for any existing or future person. One such normative theory is utilitarianism. For classic utilitarianism, what matters is maximizing aggregate utility. Since classic utilitarianism is a form of hedonistic utilitarianism, where utility translates into happiness or pleasure, the normative theory can be summarized in Jeremy Bentham's motto: "The greatest happiness for the greatest number" (Bentham, 1789/1982). Later on, Bentham refined his formulation of the utilitarian principle, arguing that the second maximization should be suppressed since it might favor the happiness of the majority at the expense of the minority. If the latter's sufferings are significant, it would not lead to maximizing happiness at all. Thus, the maximization of total happiness should be considered. In other words, the value of a state of affairs, and indirectly the appropriateness of the choice that determines that state of affairs, must be determined on an aggregate basis: utilities related to individual well-being levels for every person existing or that will exist in a given world are simply summed up to determine the world's value. According to this approach, it does not matter if additional well-being is created by improving the well-being of a particular existing or future person or by bringing into existence a non-identical but better-off person.

When applied to the Non-Identity Problem, utilitarianism seems committed to accepting what Parfit calls the No-Difference View, meaning that personal and impersonal harms are morally equivalent. Parfit asks us to consider two medical programs to detect rare diseases: if a pregnant woman has disease J, she will have a handicapped child; however, simple treatment will prevent her child from being affected. But if a woman has disease K before conceiving and still decides to proceed with her procreative project, this will lead to the birth of an individual with the same disability; disease K cannot be cured but can be prevented by delaying conception by two months. According to the No-Difference View, programs K and J are morally equivalent; therefore, if a State had to decide which programs to fund, there would be no moral reasons to choose one over the other (Parfit, 1984; Roberts, 2019). In summary, returning to Anna and Eddie's example and deeming valid impersonal harm, we can observe that the couple committed a morally wrong action by conceiving now instead of waiting three months (Singer, 2015), even if no individual has been disadvantaged by such an act.

3.2.2.1   *The Problems of the Impersonal Strategy*

The impersonal strategy as outlined, supported by a utilitarian, or other consequentialist and maximizing theory, faces various challenges. For some authors, these render such a strategy even less plausible than the Implausible Conclusion arising from the Non-Identity Problem. First, this perspective is committed to a certain form of symmetry. If we start from the assumption that the existence of an individual is a good thing when life is worth living, it follows that if it is wrong to create a life that is not worth living, then we have a moral obligation to bring about the existence of people with a life full of well-being (R. M. Hare, 1975). This has significant implications. In reproductive terms, this means using contraception is at least *prima facie* morally wrong, and giving birth to "happy" individuals is morally mandatory.

Furthermore, this approach leads to other highly counterintuitive outcomes, such as the Repugnant Conclusion. If maximizing well-being is what matters from a moral point of view, an action might increase the aggregate well-being of a population simply by increasing the number of individuals (whose lives are at least marginally worth living). This leads to the idea that a population whose members have a good quality of life could be worse than a much larger population whose members have lives that are barely worth living (Parfit, 1984). In other words, a maximizing consequentialist conception suggests that lower quality can be compensated by larger quantity. It is interesting to note that the Repugnant Conclusion, although not in these terms, had already been formulated by Henry Sidgwick in *The Methods of Ethics*:

> Assuming, then, that the average happiness of human beings is a positive quantity, it seems clear that, supposing the average happiness enjoyed remains undiminished, Utilitarianism directs us to make the number enjoying it as great as possible. But if we foresee as possible that an increase in numbers will be accompanied by a decrease in average happiness or vice versa, a point arises which has not only never been formally noticed, but which seems to have been substantially overlooked by many Utilitarians. For if we take Utilitarianism to prescribe, as the ultimate end of action, happiness on the whole, and not any individual's happiness, unless considered as an element of the whole, it would follow that, if the additional population enjoy on the whole positive happiness, we ought to weigh the amount of happiness gained by the extra number against the amount lost by the remainder.
>
> (Sidgwick, 1874/1962, p. 415)

For many, the Repugnant Conclusion is even harder to accept than the Implausible Conclusion.[18] In light of this, Parfit argues that the true challenge of moral reflection is to develop a theory, the so-called Theory X, capable of solving the Non-Identity Problem – that is, rejecting the Implausible Conclusion without leading to the Repugnant Conclusion. However, Parfit admits that he was unable to identify such a theory (1984).

To solve this *impasse*, some have argued that the underlying normative theory needs revision. Until now, utilitarianism has been considered in terms of maximizing general aggregate well-being (hence "total utilitarianism"). To avoid the Repugnant Conclusion, some authors proposed adopting "average utilitarianism", which aims to maximize not the general aggregate well-being, but the average utility of the population members (Ng, 1989). In this way, one can accept the existence of impersonal harms without falling into the Repugnant Conclusion. However, even this interpretation of utilitarianism, when applied to non-identity cases, has implications that powerfully challenge our moral intuitions. Average utilitarianism indeed implies the so-called Sadistic Conclusion (Arrhenius, 2000): assuming average utilitarianism, it is possible that adding a small number of people with a life not worth living to a given population might decrease its well-being level less than adding a large number of people with a life worth living but with well-being below the average of the given population.

Notice that, according several authors, the Repugnant Conclusion is not a knockdown argument against the impersonal strategy and should even be considered not repugnant at all (Huemer, 2008; Ryberg, 1996; Tännsjö, 2002, 2020). A common reason for this claim is that we often underestimate the quality of a life that is just above the threshold of being worthwhile. From this perspective, even those in affluent societies who enjoy privileges may lead lives just marginally over the threshold (Ryberg, 1996; Tännsjö, 2002). Defining "a life worth living" is a subject of discussion in debates on the Repugnant Conclusion. Moreover, a recent consensus paper was published among some of the most influential authors in the field of population ethics. They provide several reasons to claim that just because a theory implies a Repugnant Conclusion, it does not necessarily mean it is inadequate (Zuber et al., 2021). It is not the task of this book to discuss them. Regardless, we can still remain skeptical that morality has anything to do with an obligation to add well-being to the world, regardless of whether this has a positive impact on actual people. If a deity were to mandate the glorification of their presence through the creation of well-being in the world, this might, at least, be tenable. However, from a secular perspective, one may legitimately wonder what sort of justification there could be for a position that mandates maximizing or promoting aggregate well-being when, again, it benefits no specific individual. According to Caspar Hare, it is somewhat mysterious to assume such an obligation exists. In his words: "After all, no one can have a specific grievance against [Anna and Eddie]. Everyone can say, 'You've made things worse.' But no one can say, 'You've made things worse for me'" (C. Hare, 2007, p. 523). Therefore, anyone who rejects this possibility is also committed to rejecting the impersonal strategy.[19]

3.3 Return to the Principle of Procreative Beneficence

Based on this theoretical framework, it is now possible to clarify what it means to state that PPB is an impersonal model. Indeed, PPB assumes a conception of impersonal harm in the maximizing and consequentialist terms that are the same as those defended by the total utilitarian approach. In fact, the prescription to select the best possible child is not so much aimed at benefiting the future individual, but rather at producing a state of the world that is better than another where the selection has not taken place. Note, however, that Savulescu and Kahane do not adopt a strictly total utilitarian perspective to support PPB. Such a perspective would pre-scribe an *absolute* duty to maximize aggregate well-being through pro-creative choices, whereas this is not the case for PPB. However, while PPB generates only *prima facie* moral duties, it still does assume two features characteristic of the total utilitarian perspective: an obligation to select the best child *justified by the need* to create a world with the greatest possible well-being and a maximizing characteristic, namely, that the only moral appropriate choice is the one that maximizes the expected well-being of the future child. These two aspects are sufficient to claim that PPB shares some difficulties inherent in the utilitarian perspective.

Savulescu and Kahane might respond by arguing that PPB could be justified not only from an impersonal perspective but also from a person-affecting perspective (Savulescu & Kahane, 2009). Technically speaking, their defense is based on what Parfit called Wide Person-Affecting View (Parfit, 1984). Even assuming that the selection made by the prospective parents can harm no individual, the authors believe that, depending on genetic heritage, each embryo can benefit differently from being chosen for implantation. Thus, prospective parents should select the future child who will *benefit more* than the others by being caused to exist. In other words, by favoring the embryo with the highest expected quality of life, a greater benefit is ensured than what we might guarantee to other embryos; this greater benefit will be experienced by a specific person, i.e. the one who will exist as a result of the selection.

Rebecca Bennett effectively counters by asserting that this person-affecting interpretation of PPB ultimately falls into the impersonal con-ception: to argue that a specific child benefits more from the mere fact of being brought into the world is a genuinely impersonal argument. No person is made better or worse by the selection of embryos in the IVF plus PGD process; moreover, even assuming that existence is a benefit for the child developed from the embryo chosen by the parents (a thesis that, as we will see, is not accepted by everyone who advocates a person-affecting approach to address non-identity cases), this is the only benefit that this specific person could ever have. Thus, from the future child's perspective, talking about a greater or lesser expected benefit compared to others makes little sense. Their expected level of well-being, be it 50, 100, or 150, is, af-ter all, the only one possible for them. Therefore, if one assumes a greater benefit in giving birth to the best possible child, such a benefit would be a sort of free-floating benefit, appreciable only from a consequentialist per-spective of maximizing aggregate well-being that aims to make the world a better place from an impersonal perspective (Bennett, 2014).

Proponents of PPB ultimately recognize that the principle is not con-cerned with the benefits or harms to the resulting child. Instead, PPB asserts that it is better to give birth to a child without disabilities than to a child with a severe disability because this would make the world better in an impersonal sense (Savulescu & Kahane, 2016). This raises questions about the moral implications of understanding PPB as an impersonal principle.

3.3.1   A Principle of Reproductive Beneficence?

At this point, it is important to remark on the terminology used concerning procreative responsibility in Chapter 2: if it is clear that PPB is not concerned about the benefits or harms to the procreated child, but only about making the world a better place, and given the taxonomy proposed in Chapter 2, can this principle be considered a model or a principle of procreative-parental responsibility, or should it be considered merely a model of reproductive responsibility? Even though the moral obligations proposed by PPB are confined to the well-being of the future child, it is not possible to read such a stance within the parent–child relationship, since the parent would have no direct obligation toward the child. The duty of the reproducer would instead be to make the world a better place. Therefore, PPB should be renamed the Principle of Reproductive Beneficence.[20] Moreover, considering that PPB aims to make the world a better place, some authors argue that the principle should be modified in its formulation. In fact, according to Jakob Elster, the formulation used so far for the PPB would require too little once its fundamental theoretical assumptions are accepted. From this perspective, Savulescu proposes an unjustifiably narrow interpretation of PPB, which focuses only on the well-being of the future child. A more general understanding of the principle (Principle of General Procreative Beneficence) should be recognized:

> If couples (or single reproducers) have decided to have a child, and se-lection is possible, then they have a significant moral reason to select the child, of the possible children they could have, whose life will maximize the expected overall value in the world.
>
> (Elster, 2011, p. 483)

This formulation would clearly spell out the moral obligations of future parents in the reproductive context, which would not arise concerning their future children but the world at large.[21]

3.3.2   Procreative Beneficence and the Repugnant Conclusion

Assuming a notion of impersonal harm in maximizing and consequentialist terms, PPB would be committed to accepting the Repugnant Conclusion (Bennett, 2009, 2014). To circumvent this, Savulescu limits cases where PPB instances are valid to those where the procreative choice is a "same number choice". In other words, PPB would apply only when a couple or single reproducer decides to have a child, focusing on which child they should have. Here, PPB embraces Parfit's Q Principle: if in one of two outcomes the same number of people ever exist, it would be wrong if those living have a worse or lower quality of life than those who would have otherwise lived (Parfit, 1984, p. 360).[22] This view excludes scenarios that are judged better by totaling more benefits across a larger group of individuals. Thus, parents would not be morally obligated to reproduce and would not be committed to supporting the outcomes of the Repugnant Conclusion. In this way, PPB addresses non-identity cases without giving rise to the Repugnant Conclusion (Roberts, 2019). While intriguing, this approach seems irremediably *ad hoc* (Lillehammer, 2005; Magni, 2019). Savulescu does not give reasons to limit the principle to "same number" choices, and hence, PPB would not escape the implications of the Repugnant Conclusion, moral obligation to reproduce, or the ability to offset life quality with quantity. Consider a theoretical case where a parent must choose between having a healthy child or two asthmatic twins. PPB would commit parents to choose the asthmatic twins over the healthy child, provided the twins yield greater aggregate well-being than the single healthy child (Magni, 2021).

Supporters of the PPB might argue that, practically, procreative models will not lead to the Repugnant Conclusion. Thus, even adopting an impersonal view, PPB would not be exposed to critiques of this approach. Non-identity cases should be distinguished into two morally different categories: procreative scenarios and issues related to future generations. According to Hallvard Lillehammer, although these categories share some similarities – so much so that both Parfit and Savulescu, when defending an impersonal conception of harm, mention both procreative examples and examples related to future generations – they are quite different from a moral standpoint (Lillehammer, 2005). This is because, in reproductive cases, the potential alternative populations are too small to lead to the Repugnant Conclusion.[23] However, this reply shifts the issue from a matter of principle to one predominantly of technicality or feasibility and, therefore, fails to defend PPB effectively. Moreover, even assuming that such an argument overcomes the danger of the Repugnant Conclusion, there would still be a certain moral obligation to reproduce that not everyone, including myself, would be willing to accept.

3.3.3 Implications of a Weak Impersonal Conception: The External Challenges of Procreative Beneficence

It is worth noting that the PPB's impersonal harm conception can be defined as a weak one, which has relevant implications on how the PPB's *prima facie* instances are balanced with other reasons at play. Indeed, Savulescu and Kahane reject the No-Difference View, holding that person-affecting reasons take precedence over impersonal ones. Referring to the two genetic disease detection programs K and J, a State's decision to fund one over the other is not morally irrelevant as Parfit claims: according to PPB proponents, the State should prioritize programs offering a person-affecting benefit. In essence, actual people's concerns outweigh those of merely possible people. Regarding PPB, this means balancing the PPB and person-affecting reasons, with a certain priority given to the latter. From this perspective, PPB should be decisive mainly when no conflicting personal reasons exist.

Person-affecting reasons that need to be balanced against PPB's impersonal ones generally involve avoiding personal harm, that is, harm affecting actual people. In the selective context, the people who could suffer personal harm are not the potential children (assuming they would have a life worth living) but the mother, the couple, and other existing people in general. This highlights that if the priority is to avoid personal harm and not to produce the best possible child, it is clearer why PPB should not be seen as a model that should also be enforced by the law, undermining parents' procreative freedom. In this regard, Savulescu and Kahane refer to the concept of harm as formulated by John Stuart Mill, according to which limiting freedom is indeed personal harm, and such a limitation is justified only when the person threatens to directly and severely harm another (Mill, 1859/2003; Savulescu & Kahane, 2016). Now, since the future individual cannot be harmed when the PPB prescriptions are not pursued, the freedom of the reproducers must be protected and prioritized.

However, restricting freedom from a legal point of view is not the only personal harm at stake in the context of selective reproduction that might override PPB. As already seen in Geneva and Blake's case, in Section 3.1, undergoing an abortion might be a significant burden for the couple, and specifically for the pregnant person, precisely because the pregnant person could be harmed in many ways by the termination of pregnancy. Similarly, Savulescu and Kahane have explicitly recognized that also the psychophysical burdens of resorting to IVF might generate person-affecting reasons that can be prioritized over the PPB prescriptions. This highlights how the practical outcomes of PPB are strongly limited compared to its provocative and revolutionary theoretical contents (Ranisch, 2015). Nevertheless, according to Savulescu and Kahane, PPB would still be valid in cases where IVF is performed for other reasons, such as infertility or the risk of genetic diseases (Savulescu & Kahane, 2016).

I argue that the importance that Savulescu and Kahane give to personal harm in balancing it with the PPB's prescriptions does raise significant issues, lying in the complex definition of personal harm, which would limit PPB's practical prescriptions even more than Savulescu and Kahane might be willing to accept. Here, I no longer discuss internal challenges, seeking to criticize the principle itself, as was done in Subsection 3.1.2; rather, I focus on the PPB's external challenges, problematizing the normative scope of the principle in light of its being balanced alongside person-affecting reasons.

The concept of personal harm could be further extended in respect of what I said earlier: Savulescu and Kahane themselves argue that the loss of prospective parents' dreams, plans, aspirations, and so on could also constitute significant personal harm in the context of PPB (Savulescu & Kahane, 2016, p. 613). At this point, one might legitimately ask if sacrificing a procreator's strong desire to have a child, even if it is not the best possible child they could have, should be considered a type of personal harm inflicted on the procreator. If the answer is yes, then Savulescu and Kahane would have to admit that even if a person has already undergone IVF for infertility reasons but still deeply wishes to transfer to the uterus a "suboptimal" child, the balance between considerations should lean toward person-affecting reasons. If this is true, it would have significant implications for the practical or external normativity of the principle. Savulescu and Kahane's PPB prescriptions seem to slide toward the following:

> If a prospective parent does not desire the best possible child out of their potential children, then there is no moral obligation to select the best child because the prospective parent would be harmed in renouncing the desire not to conceive the best child. Conversely, PPB plays a significant role only if the parent is indifferent about which embryo to select or already wishes to have the best possible child.

To this, Savulescu and Kahane might respond in the following manner: claiming that person-affecting reasons are more important does not mean that PPB does not hold considerable weight and that the current generation should not make any sacrifices to prevent a significant impersonal loss of well-being in future generations (Savulescu & Kahane, 2016). However, the authors provide no tools to balance two such different types of reasons. So, there is a strong ambiguity about the strictness of the priority given to person-affecting considerations. Furthermore, no reasons are given why personal harm, even if very small, should be subordinate to impersonal harm, given the recognized priority of the former over the latter. Without satisfactory reasons to address these points, PPB would only be effective when there is no conflict between moral considerations or between the desires of the reproducers and the objectives of the PPB. Provided the putative validity of impersonal reasons, this might occur (a) when the prospective parent already wants to follow PPB or (b) when the prospective parent has no preferences about which embryo to transfer to the uterus. This would lead to the bizarre conclusion that, if there is a contrast between the reproducer's desire not to select the best possible child and the PPB prescriptions, there would be no moral reason to follow PPB rather than satisfy one's desire.

Moral duties or reasons should maintain a certain normative strength, even when confronted with personal loss endured by the agent to align with them. However, the external normativity of PPB appears to falter in this regard. It is akin to suggesting that we have to tell the truth only as long as doing so does not cause us some harm. Given that in many instances where we are inclined to lie we do so to avoid personal harm, this would imply we could abandon such a duty quite easily. But this seems implausible, as a moral obligation is actually meant to remind us that the morally appropriate action should be carried out even despite some personal cost. It seems that PPB normativity is not robust enough to consider PPB a proper generator of moral obligation. Thus, one may question the utility of establishing a moral principle that simply echoes our existing preferences or inclinations.

Notes

1 The main papers in which PPB is described and defended are Savulescu (2001, 2007, 2015) and Savulescu and Kahane (2009, 2016).

2 Remember that this statement is controversial considering the recent study already mentioned in Chapter 1 on the low efficacy of genetic selection (Karavani et al., 2019).

3 This is consistent with the Welfarist Model of Disability proposed by the same authors and discussed in Chapter 2.

4 Note that in this and the subsequent cases I will present in this book, I always refer to couples. Initially, I had framed many cases involving only a pregnant person. I then decided to modify this approach. This is not because I believe that there cannot be parenting projects carried out by a single parent, but to avoid placing too much pressure solely on the pregnant person. Clearly, as highlighted in Chapter 2 and as I will further clarify in this chapter, the major psychophysical burdens are experienced by pregnant individuals during the parental evaluation, and the final word regarding procreative decisions should be theirs. In presenting my cases, I assume that couples always fully agree and make these decisions together, making the pregnant person supported in the pregnancy journey. Moreover, it is important to clarify that in this book, I do not intend to express any moral judgment about family structures. My primary concern is with the outcomes of procreative acts themselves. I chose this approach to maintain a specific focus on the ethical considerations surrounding procreation, without delving into the diverse and complex nature of family dynamics and structures. I thank Silvia Camporesi for raising this crucial point to me.

5 Ranisch recognizes that PPB might in principle advocate for enhancement, but perhaps without radical eugenic connotations. His primary reasoning stems from empirical forecasts in genetics and genome editing. However, if rGE ever achieves an unforeseen level of safeness, precision, or efficiency, his stance might require reevaluation (Ranisch, 2022).

6 Note that my point here is not normative but merely descriptive with regard to how reproduction is perceived by Western society. I am not neglecting that in reproduction, there is always an element of public health concerns as any future child is also a future citizen (Camporesi & Cavaliere, 2018; Stern, 2005). Rather, I am simply stating that in the Western world, particularly since the aftermath of World War II, reproduction has increasingly been viewed as a private matter. This observation in itself is sufficient to contend that the critique of coercive eugenics is, at the very least, debatable without additional evidence.

7 I will discuss genetic enhancement and procreative-parental responsibility in Chapter 6.

8 I will discuss the concept of identity in procreative context in Chapter 5 (Section 5.1).

9 This example is reported in Savulescu (2001), although it is deliberately inspired by the examples of Parfit (1984).

10 For an in-depth analysis of the notion of harm, see, among others, Feinberg (1989).

11 Some argue that harm can be non-comparative, suggesting that this approach can resolve the Non-Identity Problem (Harman, 2009; Rivera-López, 2009; Shiffrin, 1999). However, this view has been extensively criticized (Boonin, 2014; Klocksiem, 2010). For the purposes of this book, I have chosen not to address this issue, since the thesis I will present in the following chapters can be defended from a comparative and intuitive notion of harm.

12 For an in-depth discussion of the Non-Identity Problem, in addition to the aforementioned texts and, in particular, the work of Parfit, see, among others, Glover (2018), Richard Mervyn Hare (1975), McMahan (2009), McMahan et al. (2022), and Narveson (1967).

13 For a complete discussion of the most important strategies proposed to solve the Non-Identity Problem, see Boonin (2014).

14 Lesch–Nyhan syndrome is a rare inherited disorder caused by a deficiency of the enzyme hypoxanthine-guanine phosphoribosyltransferase. This deficiency leads to severe neurologic dysfunction and cognitive and behavioral disturbances, including self-mutilation. A child with this condition may live into young adulthood but typically in a state of significant physical and mental distress. However, Tay–Sachs disease results in the destruction of nerve cells in the brain and spinal cord. In its infantile form, it can cause delays in mental and motor development, muscle weakness, vision problems, and, in some cases, an abnormally large head. Babies with this condition usually die by the age of 5.

15 Note that this argument, although significantly supported in the literature, is not unanimously defended. For instance, Heyd argues that not even in cases where it is foreseeable to generate a life not worth living can the comparison be considered appropriate (Heyd, 1992). I will discuss this point in Chapter 4 (Subsection 4.2.1).

16 Räsänen formulation of the *de re/de dicto* distinction may explicitly provide some further justification for PPB.

17 Some might argue, not a little controversially, that someone with a higher level of health can contribute more to the prosperity and well-being of other people.

18 The Repugnant Conclusion is not the only problem that impersonal proposals face. Think, for instance, to the Absurd Conclusion (Parfit, 1984).

19 Although only the utilitarian approach is discussed here, other approaches have been proposed in the debate. Some authors, for instance, state that not only the quantity of aggregate well-being matters but also the extent to which a state

of affairs realizes other values (Broome, 2004), such as the concept of desert (Feldman, 1995). Others rely on sufficientarism, according to which there is no maximization needed but just an obligation not to produce lives that possess less than a sufficient quality of life (Huseby, 2010). Despite the fact that these approaches do not lead to the Repugnant Conclusion, they face several challenges as well (Roberts, 2019). I have mainly discussed utilitarianism because it is useful for me in addressing PPB as an impersonal procreative responsibility model.

20 Although I think the new terminology is more appropriate, for the sake of clarity, in what follows, I will continue to use the denomination proposed by Savulescu.

21 The Principle of General Procreative Beneficence proposed by Elster is a model of impersonal reproductive responsibility. Other models of reproductive responsibility proposed in the literature are instead based on solely person-affecting reasons. I will explore the latter in Chapter 4 (Section 4.4).

22 This strategy is also adopted by the aforementioned Principle N, which, in this context, is exposed to the same critical issues as PPB (Buchanan et al., 2000) as well as the strategy proposed by Holtug (2010).

23 Zuber and colleagues argue that even in the context of population ethics, it would be implausible to hypothesize such an unrealistic situation as that envisaged by the Repugnant Conclusion (Zuber et al., 2021).

References

Adams, R. M. (1979). Existence, self-interest, and the problem of evil. *Nous, 13*(1), 53.

Anomaly, J., & Johnson, T. (2023). The ethics of genetic enhancement: Key concepts and future prospects. In F. Jotterand & M. Ienca (Eds.), *The Routledge Handbook of the ethics of human enhancement* (pp. 145–153). Routledge.

Arrhenius, G. (2000). An impossibility theorem for welfarist axiologies. *Economics and Philosophy, 16*(2), 247–266.

Benatar, D. (2006). *Better never to have been.* Clarendon Press.

Bennett, R. (2009). The fallacy of the Principle of Procreative Beneficence. *Bioethics, 23*(5), 265–273.

Bennett, R. (2014). When intuition is not enough. Why the Principle of Procreative Beneficence must work much harder to justify its eugenic vision. *Bioethics, 28*(9), 447–455.

Bentham, J. (1982). *Introduction to the principles of morals and legislation.* Law Book Co of Australasia. (Original work published 1789)

Boonin, D. (2008). How to solve the non-identity problem. *Public Affairs Quarterly, 22*(2), 129–159.

Boonin, D. (2014). *Non-identity problem and the ethics of future people.* Oxford University Press.

Bourne, H., Douglas, T., & Savulescu, J. (2012). Procreative beneficence and in vitro gametogenesis. *Monash Bioethics Review, 30*(2), 29–48.

Broome, J. (2004). *Weighing lives.* Clarendon Press.

Buchanan, A. (1996). Choosing who will be disabled: Genetic intervention and the morality of inclusion. *Social Philosophy & Policy, 13*(2), 18–46.

Buchanan, A., Brock, D. W., Daniels, N., & Wikler, D. (2000). *From chance to choice.* Cambridge University Press.

Buller, T., & Bauer, S. (2011). Balancing procreative autonomy and parental responsibility. *Cambridge Quarterly of Healthcare Ethics: CQ: The International Journal of Healthcare Ethics Committees, 20*(2), 268–276.

Camporesi, S., & Cavaliere, G. (2018). Eugenics and enhancement in contemporary genomics. In G. Sahra, B. Prainsack, S. Hilgartner, & L. Janelle. (Eds.), *Routledge Handbook of genomics, health and society.* Routledge.

de Melo-Martin, I. (2004). On our obligation to select the best children: A reply to Savulescu. *Bioethics, 18*(1), 72–83.

Dees, M. K., Vernooij-Dassen, M. J., Dekkers, W. J., Vissers, K. C., & van Weel, C. (2011). "Unbearable suffering": A qualitative study on the perspectives of patients who request assistance in dying. *Journal of Medical Ethics, 37*(12), 727–734.

DeGrazia, D. (2016). *Procreative responsibility in view of what parents owe their children* (L. Francis, Ed.). Oxford University Press.

Ehn, M., Anderzén-Carlsson, A., Möller, C., & Wahlqvist, M. (2019). Life strategies of people with deaf-blindness due to Usher syndrome type 2a – a qualitative study. *International Journal of Qualitative Studies on Health and Well-Being, 14*(1), 1656790.

Elster, J. (2011). Procreative beneficence: Cui bono? *Bioethics, 25*(9), 482–488.

Feinberg, J. (1989). *The moral limits of the criminal law: volume 1: harm to others.* Oxford University Press.

Feldman, F. (1995). Justice, desert, and the repugnant conclusion. *Utilitas, 7*(2), 189–206.

Gantsho, L. (2022). The principle of procreative beneficence and its implications for genetic engineering. *Theoretical Medicine and Bioethics, 43*(5–6), 307–328.

Glover, J. (2018). Future people, disability, and screening. In *Philosophy, politics, and society* (pp. 127–143). Yale University Press.

Hare, C. (2007). Voices from another world: Must we respect the interests of people who do not, and will never, exist? *Ethics, 117*(3), 498–523.

Hare, R. M. (1975). Abortion and the golden rule. *Philosophy & Public Affairs, 4*(3), 201–222.

Hare, R. M. (1988). Possible people. *Bioethics, 2*(4), 279–293.

Harman, E. (2009). Harming as causing harm. In M. A. Roberts & D. T. Wasserman (Eds.), *Harming future persons* (pp. 137–154). Springer Netherlands.

Harris, J. (1990). The wrong of wrongful life. *Journal of Law and Society, 17*(1), 90.

Heyd, D. (1992). *Genethics.* University of California Press.

Holtug, N. (2010). *Persons, interests, and justice.* Oxford University Press.

Hotke, A. (2014). The principle of procreative beneficence: Old arguments and a new challenge. *Bioethics, 28*(5), 255–262.

Huemer, M. (2008). In defence of repugnance. *Mind; A Quarterly Review of Psychology and Philosophy, 117*(468), 899–933.

Huseby, R. (2010). Person-affecting moral theory, non-identity and future people. *Environmental Values, 19*(2), 193–210.

Immerman, D. (2021). The worse than nothing account of harm and the preemption problem. *Journal of Moral Philosophy*, *19*(1), 25–48.

Johansson, J. (2019). The subject of harm in non-identity cases. *Ethical Theory and Moral Practice: An International Forum*, *22*(4), 825–839.

Karavani, E., Zuk, O., Zeevi, D., Barzilai, N., Stefanis, N. C., Hatzimanolis, A., Smyrnis, N., Avramopoulos, D., Kruglyak, L., Atzmon, G., Lam, M., Lencz, T., & Carmi, S. (2019). Screening human embryos for polygenic traits has limited utility. *Cell*, *179*(6), 1424–1435.e8.

Klocksiem, J. (2010). In defense of the trichotomy thesis. *Acta Analytica*, *25*(3), 317–327.

Lillehammer, H. (2005). Benefit, disability and the non-identity problem. In *Philosophical reflections on medical ethics* (pp. 24–43). Palgrave Macmillan UK.

Magni, S. F. (2019). Procreative beneficence toward whom? *Croatian Journal of Philosophy*, *19*(1), 71–80.

Magni, S. F. (2021). In defence of person-affecting procreative beneficence. *Bioethics*, *35*(5), 473–479.

McMahan, J. (2009). Asymmetries in the morality of causing people to exist. In M. A. Roberts & D. T. Wasserman (Eds.), *Harming future persons* (pp. 49–68). Springer Netherlands.

McMahan, J., Campbell, T., Goodrich, J., Ramakrishnan K., (Eds.). (2022). *Ethics and existence: The Legacy of Derek Parfit*. Oxford University Press.

Mill, J. S. (2003). *On Liberty* (G. Himmelfarb, Ed.). Penguin Classics. (Original work published 1859)

Narveson, J. (1967). Utilitarianism and new generations. *Mind; A Quarterly Review of Psychology and Philosophy*, *LXXVI*(301), 62–72.

Ng, Y.-K. (1989). What should we do about future generations? *Economics and Philosophy*, *5*(2), 235–253.

Parfit, D. (1976). On doing the best for our children. In M. D. Bayles (Ed.), *Ethics and population* (pp. 100–115). Schenkman Publishing Company.

Parfit, D. (1984). *Reasons and persons*. Oxford University Press.

Parker, M. (2007). The best possible child [Review of *The best possible child*]. *Journal of Medical Ethics*, *33*(5), 279–283. BMJ.

Ranisch, R. (2015). 'Du sollst das beste Kind wählen!'. Eine Kritik des Pflichtbegriffs von Procreative Beneficence. In R. Ranisch, S. Sebastian, & M. Rockoff (Eds.), *Selbstgestaltung des Menschen durch Biotechniken* (pp. 191–208). Francke. Verlag.

Ranisch, R. (2022). Procreative Beneficence and Genome Editing. *The American Journal of Bioethics: AJOB*, *22*(9), 20–22.

Räsänen, J. (2023). Defending the de dicto approach to the non-identity problem. *Monash Bioethics Review*, *41*(2), 124–135.

Reichlin, M. (2012). Il significato di una vita migliore. Critica al principio di beneficenza procreativa. In R. Mordacci & M. Loi (Eds.), *Etica e genetica: storia concetti e pratiche* (pp. 94–113). Mondadori.

Rivera-López, E. (2009). Individual procreative responsibility and the non-identity problem. *Pacific Philosophical Quarterly*, *90*(3), 336–363.

Roberts, M. A. (2019). Nonidentity problem. In *The Stanford Encyclopedia of Philosophy*. https://plato.stanford.edu/entries/nonidentity-problem/.

Ryberg, J. (1996). Is the repugnant conclusion repugnant? *Philosophical Papers*, *25*(3), 161–177.

Sandel, M. J. (2009). *The case against perfection*. Belknap Press.

Saunders, B. (2015). Is procreative beneficence obligatory? *Journal of Medical Ethics*, *41*(2), 175–178.

Savulescu, J. (2001). Procreative beneficence: Why we should select the best children. *Bioethics*, *15*(5–6), 413–426.

Savulescu, J. (2002). Education and debate: Deaf lesbians, "designer disability," and the future of medicine. *BMJ (Clinical Research Ed.)*, *325*(7367), 771–773.

Savulescu, J. (2007). In defence of procreative beneficence. *Journal of Medical Ethics*, *33*(5), 284–288.

Savulescu, J. (2015). Procreative beneficence, diversity, intersubjectivity, and imprecision [Review of *Procreative beneficence, diversity, intersubjectivity, and imprecision*]. *The American Journal of Bioethics: AJOB*, *15*(6), 16–18. Informa UK Limited.

Savulescu, J., & Kahane, G. (2009). The moral obligation to create children with the best chance of the best life. *Bioethics*, *23*(5), 274–290.

Savulescu, J., & Kahane, G. (2011). Disability: A welfarist approach. *Clinical Ethics*, *6*(1), 45–51.

Savulescu, J., & Kahane, G. (2016). *Understanding procreative beneficence* (L. Francis, Ed.). Oxford University Press.

Savulescu, J., Sandberg, A., & Kahane, G. (2014). Well-being and enhancement. In J. Savulescu, R. ter Meulen, & G. Kahane (Eds.), *Enhancing human capacities* (pp. 1–18). Blackwell Publishing Ltd.

Schwarz, T. (1978). Obligation to Prosperity. In R. I. Sikora, & M. B. Barry (Eds.), *Obligations to Future Generations* (pp. 3–13). Temple University Press.

Shiffrin, S. V. (1999). Wrongful life, procreative responsibility, and the significance of harm. *Legal Theory*, *5*(2). https://doi.org/10.1017/s1352325299052015

Sidgwick, H. (1962). *Methods of ethics* (7th ed.). University of Chicago Press. (Original work published 1874)

Singer, P. (2015). *Practical ethics* (2nd ed.). Cambridge University Press (Virtual Publishing).

Sparrow, R. (2007). Procreative beneficence, obligation, and eugenics. *Genomics, Society, and Policy*, *3*(3). https://doi.org/10.1186/1746-5354-3-3-43

Sparrow, R. (2011). A not-so-new eugenics. Harris and Savulescu on human enhancement. *The Hastings Center Report*, *41*(1), 32–42.

Sparrow, R. (2015). Imposing genetic diversity. *The American Journal of Bioethics: AJOB*, *15*(6), 2–10.

Steinbock, B., & McClamrock, R. (1994). When is birth unfair to the child? *The Hastings Center Report*, *24*(6), 15–21.

Stern, A. M. (2005). STERILIZED in the name of public health. *American Journal of Public Health*, *95*(7), 1128–1138.

Tännsjö, T. (2002). Why we ought to accept the repugnant conclusion. *Utilitas*, *14*(3), 339–359.

Tännsjö, T. (2020). Why Derek Parfit had reasons to accept the Repugnant Conclusion. *Utilitas, 32*(4), 387–397.

Tomlin, P. (2022). The impure non-identity problem. In J. McMahan, T. Campbell, J. Goodrich, & K. Ramakrishnan (Eds.), *Ethics and Existence: The Legacy of Derek Parfit* (pp. 93–111). Oxford University Press.

Veit, W. (2018). Procreative beneficence and genetic enhancement. *Kriterion (Salzburg), 32*(1), 75–92.

Višak, T. (2018). Engineering life expectancy and non-identity cases. *Journal of Agricultural & Environmental Ethics, 31*(2), 281–293.

Williams, N. J. (2013). Possible persons and the problem of prenatal harm. *The Journal of Ethics, 17*(4), 355–385.

Wolf, C. (2009). Do future persons presently have alternate possible identities? In *Harming future persons* (pp. 93–114). Springer Netherlands.

Zuber, S., Venkatesh, N., Tännsjö, T., Tarsney, C., Stefánsson, H. O., Steele, K., Spears, D., Sebo, J., Pivato, M., Ord, T., Ng, Y.-K., Masny, M., MacAskill, W., Lawson, N., Kuruc, K., Hutchinson, M., Gustafsson, J. E., Greaves, H., Forsberg, L., … Asheim, G. B. (2021). What should we agree on about the Repugnant Conclusion? *Utilitas, 33*(4), 379–383.

4 Person-Affecting Morality and the Future of Human Reproduction[1]

In the previous chapter, I mainly discussed impersonal, consequentialist, and maximizing approaches to guiding procreative choices. They present several problems, mainly emerging from considering impersonal reasons as valid for the moral evaluation of procreative conduct. The idea that certain acts or omissions can be harmful or wrong even when they disadvantage no actual person seems to create more difficulties than it resolves. If we consider, as proposed by the No-Difference View, person-affecting reasons morally equivalent to impersonal ones and adopt total utilitarianism, we are forced to accept the Repugnant Conclusion. If we opt for average utilitarianism, we must accept the Sadistic Conclusion. Moreover, if we adopt a weak impersonal approach that values person-affecting reasons more than impersonal ones, as suggested by Julian Savulescu and Guy Kahane, we encounter difficulty in balancing these two types of reasons, leading to the nullification of the normative force of the Principle of Procreative Beneficence (PPB). Finally, we can simply find it bizarre that morality has anything to do with an obligation to add well-being to the world, regardless of whether this has a positive impact on actual persons or at least actual sentient beings.

Due to these difficulties, some authors have proposed procreative responsibility models based only on person-affecting reasons. This chapter aims to analyze this approach, considering current Assisted Reproductive Technologies (ARTs) and, especially, future ones, particularly reproductive Genome Editing (rGE). The main focus will be on moral duties that fall within the sphere of procreative-parental responsibility; therefore, I will mainly investigate what we owe to our future children. Nonetheless, I will also devote some attention to reproductive responsibility prescriptions in order to highlight the necessity of combining these kinds of different reasons to propose a comprehensive account of procreative responsibility.

The chapter is structured as follows. In Section 4.1, I will present the consequences-based person-affecting morality and discuss some attempts to solve the Non-Identity Problem starting from this approach. In Section 4.2,

DOI: 10.4324/9781032654683-5

I will introduce one of the most discussed models of procreative-parental responsibility that has been defended from a consequences-based person-affecting perspective: the Minimum Threshold Model (MTM). I will then apply it to selective reproductive practices, like *In Vitro* Fertilization (IVF) plus Preimplantation Genetic Diagnosis (PGD). I will present and discuss one of the most insidious criticisms of this model, questioning whether a prospective parent has a truly person-affecting reason not to procreate lives not worth living. Assuming the validity of MTM in selective contexts, I will discuss whether this model also appropriately guides procreative choices in light of the availability of rGE, which will be defined as a non-identity-affecting practice. Therefore, I will introduce the Greater Moral Obligation View: given the availability of rGE, prospective parents have a greater moral obligation toward their offspring compared to what MTM requires in the context of PGD. In Section 4.3, I will explore the specific circumstances in which rGE demands an expansion of the moral obligations of future parents. Hence, I will propose two original models of procreative-parental responsibility, namely, the Bold Restriction of Procreative Autonomy and the Mild Restriction of Procreative Autonomy. Defending the latter, I will argue that new moral obligations emerge only when prospective parents have already begun the IVF process. I will claim that such a conclusion may also have relevant implications for other reproductive non-identity-affecting techniques. Finally, in Section 4.4, I will integrate procreative-parental responsibility prescriptions with two models of reproductive responsibility: Reproductive Altruism and the Principle of Generalized Reproductive Non-Maleficence.

4.1   The Consequences-Based Person-Affecting Morality

Models of procreative responsibility considering only person-affecting reasons fundamentally rest on the intuitive philosophical idea that an action or omission is morally wrong *only if* it harms someone and morally good *only if* it benefits someone (Narveson, 1973).[2] By "someone", I refer only to actual people, namely, those who have existed, exist, or will exist in the actual world (Arrhenius, 2000). From this perspective, I do not consider the interests of merely possible persons, i.e., individuals who will not exist but could have existed if different choices had been made.[3] Notice that such an approach has a peculiar focus on the consequences of procreative acts and omissions, considering only their effects and disregarding, for instance, the agent's intentions. Since, as I will argue in Chapter 7, I believe it can be reasonable to speak of person-affecting morality also considering procreative attitudes and intentions, in this chapter, I refer more specifically to this approach with the label "consequences-based person-affecting morality", bearing in mind that the label "person-affecting morality" is more commonly used in the literature. In previous papers, I attached the label "consequentialist" to the person-affecting approach assumed here (Battisti, 2021, 2023). However, I noticed that this could be misleading: such an approach can be compatible not only with consequentialist theories that aim at producing greater well-being for actual persons, but also with deontological theories that focus on rights. This is because harm can frustrate an individual's rights and opportunities.

Through this perspective, its proponents intend to resist the temptation to solve the Non-Identity Problem by theorizing impersonal harms and benefits, thus avoiding the problems discussed in the previous chapter and briefly recalled above.[4] This move can clearly have relevant and controversial implications, which have already been encountered in dealing with the Non-Identity Problem. Consider Anna and Eddie's case again: they want to have a child but discover that Anna has rubella. If they were to conceive now, their child would be born deaf and blind. If they chose to wait three months, they would conceive a healthy child. The couple decides to conceive a few days later, giving birth to a deaf-blind child. According to the consequences-based person-affecting approach, the couple's decision to bear a deaf-blind child should not be evaluated as morally wrong at all, since this choice would not harm anyone; in other terms, since morally relevant actions are only those that benefit or harm someone who exists (an actual person), deciding to produce a deaf-blind child should be considered morally permissible. Similarly, a couple undergoing IVF plus PGD does not make a morally questionable choice if they do not select the most advantaged child, as proposed by PPB. In the following subsection, I will discuss some attempts to deal with these counterintuitive consequences while still accepting consequences-based person-affecting morality.

Moreover, although this work mainly focuses on procreative choices, it is worth mentioning other and more general counterintuitive outcomes of this approach. Think, for example, of the survival and quality of life of future generations: if individuals had different identities depending on the choices others previously made, it would be morally legitimate not to care about the medium- to long-term environmental effects that a given policy might have, or to adopt a demographic policy that leads to an indiscriminate population increase. I will not discuss the Non-Identity Problem regarding collective choices, but let me advance a pragmatic defense of consequences-based person-affecting morality in these cases. One can reasonably argue that some medium- to long-term environmental policies could still be justified from this perspective. It is generally believed that the policymaker's role responsibility is to safeguard the interests of the people in a given country. These interests extend not only to the short term but also to the long term. If we acknowledge that every day new people are born in a country with an expected lifespan of 80–90 years, the policymaker should at least consider that time horizon in their decision. This argument could be taken further, albeit with weaker support, by suggesting that currently existing people genuinely want or will want in the future for their children or grandchildren, whoever they will be, not to suffer or die prematurely due to ill-advised environmental policies. In this context, the policymaker may have moral reasons to promote environmental policies that do not compromise the well-being of individuals whose identity depends on such choices, based on the interests of actual people who will have a strong emotional bond with members of future generations.

4.1.1 Consequences-Based Person-Affecting Strategies to Solve the Non-Identity Problem

As noted in the previous section, adopting a consequences-based person-affecting perspective means accepting another moral paradox, which, like the implications of impersonal theories, conflicts with common sense. Insisting that only person-affecting harms and benefits count does offer the advantage of avoiding issues like the Repugnant Conclusion or Sadistic Conclusion, but it comes at the price of *biting the bullet*, namely, accepting the Implausible Conclusion. However, various authors committed to supporting a consequences-based person-affecting approach have tried to make such a position less problematic, seeking to dodge the Implausible Conclusion; others have sought to demonstrate the plausibility of the Non-Identity Problem's implications. Regarding this latter point, an open question remains concerning how such an approach can account for the moral intuitions most people have toward the Implausible Conclusion. Below, I present some strategies that address these issues, especially regarding specific non-identity cases in the reproductive context.

4.1.1.1 The Pragmatic Strategy

To tackle the above problems, one might decide to adopt a strategy where the consequences-based person-affecting perspective is accepted, but intuitions surrounding the implausibility of the Non-Identity Problem's conclusions are accommodated. In most procreative choices, rejecting the Implausible Conclusion would be possible without adopting an impersonal approach. In this context, even though Anna and Eddie's child, who will be born deaf and blind – a condition necessary for their existence – is not harmed, one can still acknowledge that in real life, there are already existing people who are harmed by the couples' choice, such as older children or other family members (Roberts, 2009). In this case, considering the concepts introduced in Chapter 2, Anna and Eddie may have obligations from the perspective of family-based reproductive responsibility, broad reproductive responsibility, and even parental-reproductive responsibility if they have existing children who could be harmed by choosing to produce a deaf-blind child. Anna and Eddie would choose to dedicate energy, time, and money to the newcomer, sacrificing essential resources for their existing children, who could have enjoyed more resources if the couple had decided to wait three months and have a child not affected by deaf-blindness (Roberts, 2009).

This strategy is not based on a conceptual argument but a "pragmatic" one, which argues that, in actual fact, the Non-Identity Problem arises less frequently than we are led to believe. Nonetheless, even assuming the plausibility of the pragmatic argument, this does not mean there cannot be situations, at least conceptually, where the procreative choice harms no one. In these cases, resorting to the aforementioned argument to account for our intuitions regarding the Implausible Conclusion offers no explanation as to why such a conclusion remains so controversial and hard to accept for many.[5] In particular, it does not explain the intuition according to which, by giving birth immediately and not waiting three months, Anna and Eddie have done something bad *to the unborn child* – regardless of whether or not other children or people are harmed by this decision – an intuition that is resistant even if it conflicts with consequences-based person-affecting morality.

4.1.1.2 *The Genethic Strategy*

Although David Heyd also maintains that contingent facts "sting of repugnance from many of the hypothetical counterintuitive conclusions" (1992, p. 195) arising from adopting a consequences-based person-affecting approach to the Non-Identity Problem, he goes further, theorizing a more radical perspective. According to Heyd, when not "tainted" by other contextual considerations, non-identity cases do not belong to the realm of morality at all but rather to that of *genethics*. This term does not refer to genetics, understood as the branch of biology that studies genes, heredity, and genetic variability in living organisms, but rather to the genesis in a biblical sense (Singer, 1993).

Indeed, Heyd distinguishes two categories of problems: (a) "genesis" issues, or when the existence, number, and identity of future people directly depend on the choices of future parents or policymakers (e.g., procreative choices, demographic policies); and (b) issues related to how one generation takes care of the interests and quality of life of future ones (e.g., environmental issues and resource allocation).

In the latter case, the existence, identity, and number of people do not directly depend on the decision-maker but are, in fact, "given". According to Heyd, problems of type (b) could be addressed using the tools of traditional ethics, while it would not be so for problems of type (a), i.e., those that emerge from non-identity cases. Such issues are distinct because they deal with two different categories of people, namely, potential people and actual people. According to Heyd, the existence of potential persons depends on the agent's choice, which is not the case for the actual persons' existences (1992, p. 97). This means that although actual people do not necessarily exist now, they are those people who have definitely existed, exist, or will exist.

However, unlike the canonical definition according to which the actual people of the future are people whose identity is nonetheless fixed – people who will definitely exist – according to Heyd, the actual people who will live in the future have an identity that could vary. What matters is that the existence and identity of such individuals do not depend on the choice of the agent who is considering the individual's interests in their moral choice.

From this perspective, while Anna and Eddie's deaf-blind child at the time of the procreative choice was a potential child – because dependent on the couple's choice – according to Heyd, the approximately 1.7 billion people who will live in India in 2050 (Vollset et al., 2020) are actual people since their existence is already a given, at least from Anna and Eddie's point of view, even if many of them do not yet exist.

Therefore, Heyd's distinction is relative to the agent who is evaluating the moral choice: this implies that for some, a future individual will be a potential person (e.g., the parents), but for others, the same individual will be an actual person (e.g., society), and this determines different moral obligations toward the same person. Heyd proposes the example of two couples, X and Y, who are on a deserted island and cannot interfere with each other's reproductive choices. Heyd argues that the future child of couple X is a potential person for couple X, while an actual person for couple Y and vice versa. Hence, the distinction proposed here is not ontological but functional in defining the role responsibilities that the various agents of society have toward future individuals.

On the one hand, this approach would account for the fact that a policymaker, in some circumstances, has a responsibility toward future generations even from a person-affecting perspective. On the other hand, procreative choices – i.e., choices that have to do only with potential people – are not defined by Heyd as either morally right or wrong but are beyond the canonical paradigms of ethics. Such choices would belong to a non-moral deliberation sphere: the sphere of genethics. According to Heyd, bringing one or more individuals into existence and, thus, determining their identity "cannot be considered a moral problem" (Heyd, 1992, p. 126). Such decisions should be guided by a principle called Generocentrism, according to which "genesis choices can and should be guided exclusively by reference to the interests, welfare, ideals, rights, and duties of those making the choice, the 'generators,' the creators, or the procreators" (Heyd, 1992, p. 96). From this perspective, the Non-Identity Problem does not admit a *moral* resolution.

This strategy presents several flaws: the distinction between actual people and potential people proposed by Heyd, especially when considering policies and collective choices, is rather blurred. It is difficult to imagine that collective choices do not influence parents' reproductive decisions and, therefore, that the existence of future people does not also depend on these choices. The example of the deserted island does not justify the problematic assumption that couple X cannot interfere in the reproductive decisions of couple Y and vice versa: collaboration and interdependence between couples, for example, could create the conditions for one of the two couples to be able or unable to reproduce. Hence, this would influence the couple's choices about whether, when, and how much to procreate. Heyd himself argues that this distinction is difficult to trace in practical situations and that "genethics works only under idealized conditions" (Heyd, 1992, p. 24).[6]

Jeff McMahan offers further arguments to challenge the distinction between potential people and actual people proposed by Heyd. Suppose that the existence of a person Q depends on the choice of agent Z. By hypothesis, Q is for Z a potential person who, according to Heyd, Z cannot consider in their moral deliberation. Suppose, however, that the choice that Z makes brings Q into existence. In that case, Heyd's distinction between actual and potential people forced Z to ignore the interests of someone who became actual, and this would violate the assumption that all those who are at some point actual count (McMahan, 1994). This leads to rather counterintuitive outcomes in relation to cases of prenatal injuries: it would be difficult to explain, for example, that the use of drugs or alcohol in pregnancy by the mother is morally problematic because it is harmful to the future child.

Finally, like the pragmatic strategy, the genethic strategy does not provide a satisfactory explanation of why the conclusion of the Non-Identity Problem – which arises from accepting the premise that in procreating, no person is harmed – is so counterintuitive. If procreative choices are not moral at all, why do we have these strong intuitions? In other words, no reasons are offered for why the Implausible Conclusion remains controversial and difficult to accept in cases without harm to third parties.

4.1.1.3 *The Preferences Strategy*

A possible solution to the question left by the two previous strategies is offered by Rebecca Bennett, who maintains that the intuitions people feel are not properly moral but rather mere personal preferences. If it is true that

Eddie and Anna's choice does not harm anyone, then this choice is outside the realm of morality: it is a morally neutral choice, a preference, and therefore permissible (Bennett, 2009). This does not mean that Eddie and Anna cannot have good reasons to choose to wait to procreate or prefer the idea of a society containing particular types of people. However, these reasons would not be moral reasons, but simply preferences.

This explanation, however, can be challenged if we acknowledge that not all of our moral intuitions are reducible to what we prefer. In this regard, Peter Herissone-Kelly proposes the following example: suppose that in the future, PGD can reveal the IQ of future individuals and that a couple of individuals with average intelligence undergo IVF, thus producing two embryos.[7] After the PGD analysis, it was found that one embryo has average intelligence, while the other embryo has intelligence far above average. Let us assume, not without controversy,[8] that greater intelligence increases the well-being of the individual and that the parents are supporters of PPB. In light of this, it would be perfectly plausible that the parents might prefer a child with intelligence that is more similar to theirs but still feel morally obliged to select the embryo with a higher expected IQ (Herissone-Kelly, 2012).

4.1.1.4 *The Plausibility of the Implausible Conclusion*

The last strategy I consider is proposed by David Boonin. According to him, the acceptability of the Implausible Conclusion should not be sought in harm to third parties, nor in acknowledging that procreative choices are outside the scope of ethics. The pragmatic and genethic strategies appear to be mere forms of evasion designed to avoid the question (Boonin, 2008). Boonin argues that the answer to the Non-Identity Problem is clearly intelligible from a moral point of view. Indeed, the counterintuitiveness of the conclusion is only apparent; upon closer inspection, the conclusion is shareable and reasonable. From this perspective, the non-identity issue no longer appears as a real problem but as an argument (Boonin, 2008, 2014) or a principle (Weinberg, 2013).

This strategy is based on the idea that, once all the premises of the Non-Identity Problem are accepted, we should also accept its conclusion without further considering it implausible. And this does not imply considering the choice neither right nor wrong, thus rendering it morally unjudgeable, as Heyd suggests. Instead, it recognizes that choices such as the one taken by Eddie and Anna are morally appropriate and permissible choice:

> Regardless of whether we call the question an ethical one, a "genethical" one, or something else, the question of whether or not [Anna] is doing something that she ought not to do seems to be a perfectly

intelligible one and one that should have a meaningful answer. There seems, then, to be no way to resist the argument's premise, no way to resist the move from the premises to the conclusion, and no justification for simply avoiding this issue.

(Boonin, 2008, p. 144)

Boonin argues that the process of revising our moral intuitions concerning the Non-Identity Problem is no different from the approach adopted in other moral controversies: many people, for example, find it extremely implausible to claim that a six-week-old human embryo has the same right to life as an adult human being. Many have the same reaction to the statement that eating a hamburger is morally impermissible. But if a compelling argument emerged in defense of one of these claims and if, after careful examination of the argument, no flaws were found, it would be more reasonable to simply accept the conclusion of the argument rather than continue to reject it merely because initially it was thought that its conclusion was wrong (Boonin, 2014).

Furthermore, Boonin does offer an explanation for why most people find the conclusion of the Non-Identity Problem counterintuitive without appealing to the distinction between moral reasons and preferences as proposed by Bennett. He argues that people's basic moral beliefs include the belief that it is *prima facie* wrong to act in ways that significantly harm other people. Generally, an act that leads a person to have a severe disability, such as deaf-blindness, is an act that significantly harms that person. This is because an act that causes a person to have a disability makes them significantly worse off than they would otherwise have been. When our moral intuitions register disapproval of an act that implies someone has a significant disability, it is because intuition reflects this more fundamental moral belief (Boonin, 2008).

4.1.2 Adopting Consequences-Based Personal-Affecting Morality

Assessing whether the consequences-based personal-affecting approach provides a satisfactory argument for solving the Non-Identity Problem encompasses a notably complex and intricate issue. It is not the specific task of this book to delve deeply into this. Instead, I limit myself to claiming that the consequences-based person-affecting approach possesses reasonable intuitive strength, and its prescriptions – although, as we will see later for the selective ARTs, rather minimal – are capable of garnering greater consensus compared to impersonal approaches. Even Savulescu and Kahane, while proposing an impersonal principle, acknowledge the value of person-affecting reasons in procreative choices, considering them a priority.

In what follows, I aim to *provisionally* propose a discussion on consequences-based person-affecting reasons in the procreative context in light of the development of ARTs. Therefore, the goal of this reflection is not so much to argue that morality should be concerned *solely* with consequences-based personal-affecting harms and benefits, but rather to develop an argument that might be accepted by people with diverse moral conceptions, who nonetheless agree that at least consequences-based person-affecting considerations should morally constrain our actions and omissions. Considering only reasons of this type will also allow us to avoid problems that arise from the balancing of reasons of different kinds when they conflict, which, as seen in the previous chapter, Savulescu and Kahane problematically attempted to do with personal and impersonal reasons with regard to PPB (Savulescu & Kahane, 2016).

4.2   The Minimum Threshold Model

A procreative-parental responsibility model that is generally considered compatible with such a theoretical approach is MTM. According to this model:

> Every reproductive choice is legitimate except bringing children into the world when there are good reasons to think that their quality of life will fall below an acceptable threshold. This threshold separates lives worth living from those not worthy of being lived.[9]

In other words, procreating children with expected suffering that makes their lives not worth living is the only thing that is morally wrong. In the field of genetic selection via IVF and PGD, this implies that couples or single reproducers may use this technique to select embryos with specific characteristics, provided that it is not expected that the resulting child will have a life not worth living. As a consequence, this model considers morally legitimate reproductive decisions in cases where procreators, for whatever reasons, select one or more embryos not only to avoid some disability or genetic condition but even to have a child with a certain disability or specific genetic condition (Stramondo, 2017). As already mentioned in Chapter 1, although in very limited numbers, some clinics do provide or have provided this service in the past, accessed primarily by couples or reproducers with a condition generally considered a disability, who want to have a child who shares their experience, or because of personal or cultural value they placed in their genetic lineage, including the condition. In this light, it is again possible to mention the paradigmatic case of Sharon Duchesneau and Candy McCullough, even though technically the couple in question did not use PGD to have a child with deafness but rather chose sperm donation from a donor with a family history of deafness.

From this, it is easy to observe that MTM is a particularly permissive model toward the choices of future parents; as argued in the previous chapter, conditions of a life not worth living are generally considered extremely rare, leaving a wide range of choices to the parents. In this regard, MTM perfectly overlays the aforementioned Principle of Procreative Autonomy proposed by John Robertson, according to which society members would have the right to freely choose how, when, and where to reproduce (Robertson, 1994). Although this formulation does not seem to leave room for what procreators owe to their future children, Robertson still maintains that parents have at least a minimal moral duty not to procreate in order to produce children with lives that are not worth living, since "in such case existence itself is a wrong" (Robertson, 1994, p. 75).

Assume that in the future, a large number of characteristics of the future individual can be known in advance and that PGD allows a choice between several embryos. According to MTM, reproducers will be able to choose among all possible combinations freely, provided that they select an embryo whose life is expected to be worth living. In fact, according to Bennett, an MTM advocate, PGD could legitimately be used not only to select embryos that are not predisposed to develop genetic diseases – the main reason for which such practice is used today – but also to select embryos from which will develop individuals who are "deaf, hearing, 'ugly', dyslexic, short, tall, highly intelligent, etc." (Bennett, 2009, p. 271).

Once we assume MTM clears the field of putative moral duties toward future children, other morally relevant aspects remain in play in the context of procreative choices, such as the need to protect the procreative freedom of prospective parents. As a matter of fact, we can observe that MTM is also superimposable to the legal model already outlined by Savulescu for the regulation of procreative choices, according to which it would be appropriate to ensure the broadest possible freedom, as long as the life created is worth living. The clear difference between the two approaches is that, while Savulescu considers the legal model insufficient to account for the moral aspects of procreative choice, it would perfectly coincide with the moral proposal of MTM.

MTM can have significant implications not only in the PGD context but also for other ARTs discussed in Chapter 1. MTM implies a moral duty to undergo genetic carrier testing to avoid procreating a life with a genetic condition that reasonably makes the life of the future child not worth living. Furthermore, MTM could also have relevant implications in relation to prenatal testing: one could indeed argue that parents who undergo prenatal testing and find out that their future child will have a life not worth living have a moral duty to abort. While this conclusion is logically consistent, before endorsing it, one should consider the moral implications of the more significant psycho-physical burdens for the pregnant persons and the couple compared to the preimplantation scenario. Moreover, the feasibility of performing prenatal testing implies that the embryo has already been transferred *in utero*. In light of this, some people might note a difference between the moral status of the post-implantation embryo and the *in vitro* embryo. In what follows, the focus will be mainly on early embryos and ARTs, although there will be a brief mention of the moral duties of parents in the context of *in utero* genetic treatments and fetal therapy in Subsection 4.4.3.

4.2.1 *Do We Really Have a Duty to Not Generate a Life Not Worth Living?*

MTM in selective contexts is defended by several supporters of consequences-based person-affecting morality (Battisti, 2021; Bennett, 2009, 2014; Buller & Bauer, 2011; Gavaghan, 2007; Magni, 2021). Yet, is this model really consistent with such an approach? In this regard, I discuss an issue already partially addressed in Subsections 3.2.1.1 and 3.2.1.2, assessing whether prospective parents have the moral duty to avoid procreating lives not worth living. Consider the following case:

> Alex and Veronica, a 39-year-old woman with primary infertility, decide to have a child and undergo the IVF process. Although Veronica is a healthy carrier of the HPRT1 gene mutation, she opts for PGD to identify not only chromosomal anomalies, but also embryos that might develop into children affected by Lesch-Nyhan Syndrome (LND). However, due to the limited number of oocytes Veronica can produce, it is discovered that no embryos are available for transfer, except for one male embryo affected by the HPRT1 gene mutation. This mutation would lead the future individual to develop LND. Despite this, Veronica and Alex request the transfer of this embryo. Alex and Veronica deeply desire to become parents and believe this might be their last opportunity. The couple acknowledges that their future child's life could be filled with suffering but are committed to providing care.

In the previous chapter, I argued that having LND could reasonably make life not worth living. Although this statement does not meet with unanimous agreement, I assume that the couple's child, if they came into the world, would reasonably have a life not worth living.

To analyze this case, let us once again consider the account proposed by Heyd. He argues that if we accept that a child cannot be harmed by being born with a congenital disability, then there is no reason why this argument should not extend to cases where a child's life is not worth living. From

Heyd's view, adopting a consequences-based person-affecting perspective not only makes it acceptable to bring into the world a child with a disability that still allows for a meaningful life (like deafness[10] or Trisomy 21), but also to cause the existence of a child with a far more severe condition like LND.

Heyd believes non-existence is not a "state" a person can be in (Heyd, 1992, p. 30). This means we cannot compare existence against non-existence, since non-existence cannot be given any value and it is not a state that can be attributed to a subject. According to Heyd, embracing a consequences-based person-affecting morality means that even generating a life that might not be considered worth living is not morally wrong. This view is based on the idea that harm, as already claimed in Chapter 3, is comparative in nature. Therefore, when we are causing a person to exist, it would make no sense to talk about harm and benefit because the relevant alternative for evaluating such a condition in comparative terms is non-existence. Thus, there is nothing to compare. From this perspective, the MTM's prescription to avoid bringing forth "unworthy lives" seems to be a baseless or *ad hoc* argument (Ranisch, 2020).

In the same direction, McMahan argues that consequences-based person-affecting morality implies that procreative choices must assume the Individual-Affecting Symmetry (McMahan, 2009, p. 60). According to this perspective, there is complete moral symmetry between generating people with a life worth living and creating people with a life not worth living. The consequences-based person-affecting view is committed to holding that an act or an omission can be wrong only if there is a person who exists at some point in the present or future who is worse off because of that act or omission. Nevertheless, making a person exist with a miserable life cannot make them worse off, because "worse" implies a comparison with an alternative scenario that would be better for the same individual. However, the relevant alternative scenario is simply not to make them exist; in this case, however, there will never be anyone for whom non-existence is better than existence with a life not worth living, since it is decided not to make them exist. Therefore, unless the effects of the procreative choice on already existing or anyhow actual people are considered, there is moral indifference regarding the procreation of a life worth or not worth living. In sum, both McMahan and Heyd support something we may call *noncomparability*.

At first glance, some may try to reject McMahan's and Heyd's position arguing that this strong noncomparability implies that painlessly killing a person would not constitute a morally wrong act: in fact, death, a condition of non-existence, does not make the individual killed worse off than previously since non-existence is incomparable with existence. Furthermore, according to Thomas Petersen, it is incorrect to argue that to define a person as better or worse off (in existential terms), we necessarily need to compare two states of affairs in which the person exists. To prove this, he imagines two worlds: World 1, where Alison has lived for 30 years and so far has had a good life, a life that has contained more well-being than suffering, and World 2, where Alison will never exist. It is evident that Alison, if rational, should prefer World 1 because this alternative could better satisfy her interest (Petersen, 2001).

The supporters of noncomparability reject this reply. They argue that in both cases of homicide and Alison, there is already an actual person who suffers or would suffer from the cessation of their existence. This cannot be the case in the procreative context, where the person who might have a life not worth living would never exist, in light of the MTM obligation not to generate lives not worth living. A person who does not exist cannot have interests; therefore, the two scenarios would not be morally analogous. In Heyd words, "only death can be attributed as a loss to a person – not the state of never being conceived" (Heyd, 1992, p. 31).

In light of this clarification, we have a complete argument here. Therefore, assuming its plausibility, we can ask what the implications of noncomparability are for MTM. It seems to me that two options are open: (a) rejecting the consequences-based person-affecting perspective and claiming that this theoretical framework cannot support MTM and, therefore, referring to some – problematic – impersonal perspective. In a similar direction, McMahan claims that, in light of the noncomparability, the moral wrong in procreating lives not worth living can only have an impersonal explanation; (b) alternatively, we can keep the consequences-based person-affecting perspective and reject MTM, arguing that it is legitimate to procreate lives not worth living, a perspective in open contrast with commonsense morality. In this case, to remove the sting from this terrible conclusion, it can be argued that there is a moral imperative to consider the option of euthanasia or to provide compassionate end-of-life care from the very beginning of the child's life. Nevertheless, it would sometimes not be possible to end the existence of people whose lives would be overwhelmed by suffering before they have experienced severe torment; this would again push us to support a moral duty not to generate lives not worth living, forcing us to reconsider a procreative responsibility taking into account impersonal reasons to justify this duty (McMahan, 2009).

I claim that noncomparability is not as obvious a position as its supporters believe. If this perspective can be reasonably rejected, there might be a good chance of saving MTM without giving up the consequences-based person-affecting perspective. Therefore, I propose some strategies below that can do this. The debate on the issue is complex; thus, I present only three strategies that can reasonably be evaluated without necessarily leaning toward one or the other.

The first strategy argues that the term "existence" in this debate is ambiguous and often seems to presuppose that people coming to exist are like the light of a lamp that turns on with a click of a switch. Nonetheless, in line with David DeGrazia, we can note that, before becoming a person, an individual may have begun to exist as a fetus or an embryo (DeGrazia, 2016). In other words, an individual may start to exist well before birth as a numerical identity, not necessarily as a being endowed with moral status. Therefore, even conceding the noncomparability between existence and non-existence – meaning existence in the sense of starting to exist as a numerical identity and not as a birth – we can still defend MTM from a consequences-based person-affecting perspective. From this perspective, the embryo affected by the HPRT1 gene mutation produced by Alex and Veronica, which cannot currently feel pain, should not be transferred into the uterus. Likewise, a couple who discovers during pregnancy that a fetus has a condition that reasonably makes future life not worth living may be aborted before beginning a life overwhelmed by suffering. In these two cases, "the charge of wrongful life, then, applies not necessarily to the creation of the life in question but to the decision to allow it to continue beyond the presentient stage of life during which suffering is impossible" (DeGrazia, 2016, p. 643). This strategy is appealing and elegantly manages to escape the pitfalls of noncomparability without being committed to comparability between existence and non-existence. However, it should be noted that it relies on a challenging assumption, which I will discuss in Chapter 5: we come into existence as human organisms long before we acquire any mental state (DeGrazia, 2016). Authors who think that we are, say, embodied minds could not accept this perspective on identity, but this – as I will discuss – comes at the price of accepting other controversial claims.

The second strategy consists, instead, of directly rejecting noncomparability and arguing that a comparison can be made. Melinda A. Roberts argues that non-existing people can be attributed a welfare value, namely, 0, which can increase when brought into the world with a life worth living and decrease if born with a life not worth living (Roberts, 2003). Moreover, she responds to the argument that in the case of avoiding procreating lives that are not worth living, there would be no subject. Similar to the aforementioned case of Alison, Roberts argues that each of us can imagine a scenario in which we are 100 years old and seriously ill and wonder whether continuing to exist is worse than dying. This means hypothesizing that well-being could continue to decline if we exist, while it could stop decreasing if we no longer exist: "if [we] go out of existence, [we] will incur no further burdens and accrue no further benefits" (Roberts, 2011a, 769). Roberts proposes a comparison between this scenario and a procreative one and argues that a comparison between existence and non-existence is possible in both since, in both scenarios, we are still dealing with a subject. Roberts recognizes that the subject does not exist in the world in which prospective parents choose not to bring into existence a person with an unworthwhile life; in the same way, we do not continue to exist in the world in which we choose to terminate our life. But since the future could have developed in a way that encompassed the child with a life not worth living, just as the future could have unfolded in a manner that (still) includes us with 100 years old and severely ill (Roberts, 2011a), in both cases there is still a subject. From this perspective, it is a matter of considering a possible world in which a person who does not exist now will exist and experience such suffering as to prefer non-existence to existence.

Although the strategy of attributing to the non-existence 0 welfare value received some support (Bradley, 2013; Feit, 2016), it is not free from controversy: Christian Piller recently stated, for example, that we cannot claim to enjoy a higher level of well-being in our existence than if we had never existed because we do not reach any level of well-being if we fail to exist (Piller, 2023).[11] Here, I just notice that accepting Roberts' perspective would save MTM since the notion of comparative harm we consider in this work applies perfectly to cases of existence/non-existence: a person who does not exist should be assigned a well-being value of 0; if this person came into the world with a life not worth living, their well-being would be negative and, therefore, they would be in a state worse than non-existence. This person would then be harmed in a comparative sense by existing.

Finally, the third strategy suggests framing existence against non-existence not in terms of worse and better but rather in terms of *good* and *bad* (Parfit, 1982, 1984). From this perspective, it may be conceded that causing someone to exist with a life not worth living cannot be worse for that person. However, this life can still be bad for them, that is, *worse than nothing*. Therefore, good reasons would emerge to prevent a child with a life not worth living from experiencing this existential bad. This life would be bad for the child. This reason would be explainable from a consequences-based person-affecting perspective, similar to the previous strategy. Nonetheless, there is a substantial difference between this and the previous strategy: while previously it was possible to refer to comparative harm, in this case, we need to appeal to a non-comparative notion of harm. Unlike other versions already mentioned in the previous chapter (Note 12, Chapter 3), such a notion applies only in existential circumstances, when a person comes into the world exhaustively predetermined, making it impossible to pursue all current and future goals, whatever they may be.[12]

The three strategies presented seem to effectively defend the moral obligation not to procreate lives not worth living from a consequences-based person-affecting perspective. However, if we focus on the second and the third strategies, another crucial problem might arise: some could argue that the second strategy – claiming that non-existence can be better than a life not worth living – is committed to arguing that a life worth living is *better* than non-existence, thus, a benefit. In other words, if being alive can be worse than not being born at all, it can be better too (Roberts, 2011a). With regard to the third strategy, since a life not worth living constitutes an existential non-comparative harm to the person who exists, a happy and worthwhile life constitutes an *existential non-comparative benefit*. This seems to provide beneficence person-affecting reasons to generate lives worth living (Roberts, 2011a). From this perspective, having a moral duty not to create a life not worth living implies a duty to reproduce because, in doing so, we would be producing a benefit or a good to a person who exists. But this resembles one of the conclusions that have reasonably led us to abandon the impersonal approach to procreative choices.

In other words, for MTM to be defensible, it is not enough to justify the claim that it is wrong to produce a child whose existence is not worth living. It should also be avoided being committed to claiming a duty to produce lives worth living. In other words, MTM must be compatible with the so-called Asymmetry,[13] according to which (a) it is wrong to bring a child with a life not worth living into existence but (b) permissible not to bring a child with a life worth living into existence. However, several authors maintain that the Asymmetry is untenable (McMahan, 2009; Persson, 2009; Singer, 2015; Sprigge, 1968) and that assuming the consequences-based person-affecting perspective implies, instead, a *symmetry of obligations*: if there is no moral duty to create lives worth living, there is no duty to avoid creating lives unworthy of living either; if instead there is a duty to refrain from creating lives not worth living, then there is also a duty to reproduce with the specific aim to generate lives worth living.

At this point, we might note that it would be enough to embrace the first strategy discussed and to be able to accept both (a) and (b) without much trouble. But here I intend to provide arguments to accept both (a) and (b) even by embracing either the second strategy or the third strategy. To do this, some may appeal to the alleged distinction between harms and benefits according to which avoiding harm has moral precedence over producing a benefit; I do not follow this path.[14] I suggest, instead, that if what counts are only benefits and harm to actual people, then we are not committed to claiming that there is a moral duty to bring to the existence a child with a life worth living. To justify this, I propose a simple test consisting of assessing what would happen if an agent violated the two moral obligations that critics consider symmetric in light of the plausibility of the second and the third strategies: (i) the duty not to bring into the world an unworthwhile life; and (ii) the duty to reproduce in order to create a child with a life worth living who can be said to be in a better state than non-existence or simply to be in a good state. If the agent violates (i), then an actual person will exist and experience overwhelming suffering. In contrast, if one contravenes (ii), no actual person will suffer, and no actual person will be able to express complaints for the missed benefit or good. Only when we consider (i) the agent commits a person-affecting harm, and this provides strong moral reasons to avoid causing suffering to an existing person. Conversely, not procreating does not affect any actual person; hence, it cannot be objectionable from the consequences-based person-affecting standpoint assumed in this chapter.[15]

Of course, the discussion could continue, but what has been said seems enough to argue that MTM can reasonably be justified in the consequences-based person-affecting perspective assumed in this chapter and, therefore, that this model should guide procreative choices in selective contexts like that of IVF plus PGD.[16] With this, there would be good reasons to argue that Alex and Veronica have a moral duty not to transfer the embryo affected by LND.

However, in addition to the theoretical problems discussed in these pages, we should notice again that MTM is certainly not free from controversy, which, as argued in Chapter 3, is mainly related to the fact that it is difficult, if not impossible, to provide a clear and non-arbitrary line that divides all cases of worthy lives from cases of lives not worth living; with this in mind, Jonathan Glover defines such a threshold "largely a philosopher's abstraction" (Glover, 2006, p. 57). Subsequently, I will discuss whether or not this model is appropriate to inform procreative choices in light of the future possibility of modifying the human genome.

4.3   The Minimum Threshold Model and Genome Editing

So far, I have analyzed MTM within the context of PGD, developing some theoretical considerations aimed at justifying its prescriptions in selective contexts. Since PGD involves selecting between several embryos, this technique neither harms nor wrongs any individual, except in cases where an embryo is selected with an expected quality of life that makes the future child's life not worth living. Therefore, PGD typically does not affect the person[17]; thus, I consider genetic selection occurring after IVF via PGD an identity-affecting procedure.

In this section, assuming the validity of MTM in selective contexts, I will evaluate whether rGE has different moral implications compared to PGD. In other words, I intend to assess whether MTM is an appropriate tool to guide reproductive choices also in light of the future availability of rGE. Although human genetic modification has been central to the bioethical debate in past decades, recent technological developments presented in Chapter 1 indicate that rGE could reasonably be considered safe for use in human reproduction soon. This has renewed attention on the relationship between rGE and person-affecting morality (Alonso & Savulescu, 2021; Battisti, 2021, 2023; Cavaliere, 2018; Feeney & Rakić, 2021; McMahan & Savulescu, 2023; Palacios-González, 2021; Ranisch, 2020; Rulli, 2019; Savulescu & Alonso, 2022; Schaefer, 2020; Sparrow, 2022).

At first glance, we can notice the similarities between rGE and PGD from the viewpoint of the reproducers: both practices can be used in IVF to transfer embryos that will have specific traits according to the parents' preferences. However, while PGD performs merely selective action on embryos, rGE enables the modification of a particular embryo instead, which may have morally relevant consequences. If we assume that the modified embryo shares the *numerical identity* with the future individual,[18] such a genetic modification may lead to significant effects on the future individual who will develop from the modified embryo. In other words, intervening in the genetic heritage of an embryo before it is transferred into the uterus could harm or benefit a specific person who will surely exist. Likewise, refraining from using rGE ensures that a specific individual is in a worse or better condition than if the modification had taken place.

From this, I argue that an embryo's genome is no longer beyond the parents' control: thanks to the future availability of rGE, an embryo will have a series of possibilities, namely, different versions of its genome, with which to come into existence. In this context, we are no longer dealing with a choice between "existence" or "non-existence", as in the case of PGD; instead, we are choosing to change the genetic heritage of the future individual, which would have been qualitatively different without such modification, or with a different modification. Modifying the genome of an embryo affected by a particular genetic condition will cause this embryo to develop into a numerically identical child who, without genome modification, would have suffered from a genetic disease (Omerbasic, 2018). In light of this, it is reasonable to define rGE as a *non-identity-affecting practice*, unlike PGD.[19] In some previous papers, I referred to rGE with the term "person-affecting technique" or "person-affecting procedure" (Battisti, 2021, 2023), in line with other authors (Ranisch, 2022; Sparrow, 2022). Although these terms are not incorrect, in this book, I use the label "non-identity affecting practice" to minimize conceptual confusion. I will apply "person-affecting" when referring to harms, benefits, reasons, or moral perspectives that contrast with impersonal ones. "Non-identity-affecting" will be used, instead, to describe actions, choices, or technology that do not change the numerical identity of the individuals involved, as opposed to those that are "identity affecting".[20] Clearly, the terms are related but not interchangeable. For example, an action that does not affect the identity of the individual involved may give rise to person-affecting moral reasons to perform or not to perform that action. Conversely, an action that affects the identity of the person will not generate new person-affecting moral reasons.

At this point, a question arises: what is entailed by conceiving rGE as a non-identity-affecting procedure? I argue that this commits us to accept the Greater Moral Obligation View, namely, the thesis that the availability of rGE generates new moral obligations toward progeny, even accepting the very weak constraints on procreative freedom in the field of PGD and other selective ARTs proposed by MTM. To make my point clear, I present two thought experiments: the case of Julia and that of Jeff-to-be (Battisti, 2021):

Julia's case

Julia is a newborn who is affected by disease X, which, though not so severe as to make her life not worth living, is likely to significantly compromise either: (a) her physical or psychological well-being; or (b) her range of opportunities for choosing her own life plan; or (c) the possibility to develop abilities and skills necessary to pursue a reasonable range of those opportunities and alternatives; or (d) the capacities for practical reasoning and judgment that enable the individual to engage in reasoned and critical deliberation about those choices.

It is reasonable to argue that a significant impairment of (a)–(c) and/ or (d) amounts to harming Julia. Therefore, I assume we will encounter a broad consensus among people if we consider X harmful to Julia and, consequently, if we claim that Julia's parents have a *prima facie* moral duty to cure her of X, provided that cure Y is available, effective, safe, legal, and cheap. In these circumstances, parents would have *control* over Julia's state of health; therefore, if they refuse to cure her, Julia could reasonably complain about her parents' decisions. If, on the contrary, Julia were affected by an untreatable disease Z, it would be hard to claim that her parents are responsible for Julia's state of health: in this case, Julia could not complain about her condition to her parents because a cure for Z does not exist. While the parents have a moral obligation to cure Julia of X, the same does not hold for Z, since moral duties strictly depend on the parents' capabilities to cure Julia, which rely on the technological possibilities, the affordability of the treatments, etc. In fact, as I have argued, the role of responsibility parents face in these circumstances depends on the material capacity of the parents.

Let us now consider another scenario:

Jeff-to-be's case

Jeff-to-be is an *in vitro* embryo about to be implanted in his mother's uterus to develop into a person called Jeff. Jeff-to-be is affected by a genetic mutation causing a genetic disease X_1, which is likely to impair his physical or psychological well-being and/or curtail the reasonable range of opportunities in the same way as X affected Julia. As in Julia's case, Jeff's life with X_1 is expected to be worth living. A rGE treatment Y_1 that solves the genetic mutation leading to X_1 is available, effective, safe, legal, and cheap. However, the prospective parents decide to transfer Jeff-to-be without modifying his genome and, as a consequence, after 9 months Jeff is born affected by X_1.

Although this scenario may seem unrealistic for many people, it may occur for several reasons: here I present some of them in a range from the most unlikely to the most plausible ones. First, Jeff-to-be's parents have sadistic personalities, and they want to bring into the world a child who suffers from genetic disease X_1.[21] Second, his parents might want to have a sick child to take care of him for his whole life. Third, the parents-to-be believe that X_1 is not a condition that cuts off opportunities for Jeff; on the contrary, they think that X_1 may help him interact with a specific community to which the parents belong. Finally, the prospective parents do not know about Jeff's genetic condition, since they did not engage in any process of genetic screening of the embryo to detect genetic diseases of Jeff-to-be. This last scenario seems plausible considering that, according to the 2020 Assisted Reproductive Technology Fertility Clinic Success Rates Report mentioned in Chapter 1, about 48% of IVF cycles reported the transfer of at least one embryo that underwent preimplantation genetic testing during 2020 in the United States. Regardless of whether the case of the Jeff-to-be is realistic or not, it is particularly helpful for understanding whether there are and what moral duties emerge from the future availability of rGE.

Although in Julia's case, the existence of a moral duty to care for the newborn is particularly noncontroversial, the moral evaluation in Jeff's case may not be so immediate. To assess whether the Jeff-to-be's parents committed a morally wrong act, I propose a comparison between Julia's case and that of future Jeff, in order to verify whether there are any morally relevant analogies. At first glance, we notice that both treatments Y and Y_1 are available, effective, cheap, legal, and safe. Second, Julia and Jeff would both be harmed, respectively, by X and X_1, should the parents decide not to treat with Y and Y_1: in both cases, the parents' decision affects their respective child, already existing in Julia's case, or future, in Jeff's case. Both Julia and Jeff have a right to complain about their parents' decisions.[22] In light of this, there seem to be good reasons to argue that parents have a *prima facie* moral duty to treat Jeff-to-be with Y_1. Indeed, the moral reasons that, in Julia's case, give rise to the duty to treat her with Y also arise in the case of future Jeff. Therefore, if we accept that in Julia's case, the parents have a moral obligation to treat the newborn, then we are also committed to accepting the existence of a moral duty to treat Jeff-to-be with rGE.[23]

Having established the moral similarity between the cases of Jeff-to-be and Julia, we should explore how the limits of procreative-parental responsibility effectively shift and under what circumstances parents face greater moral obligations toward their offspring. But before proceeding with this, clarification is needed. In Julia's case, her parents are facing two options: (a) to cure her or (b) not to cure her, and only the former should be considered morally legitimate. Conversely, in Jeff-to-be's case, the parents-to-be face three options because we are not dealing with a person yet.[24] Even though I argued that rGE is non-identity affecting, it does not mean that the embryo is already a person with full moral status at the time of modification. Rather, the actions performed on that embryo will affect a future individual endowed with full moral status. Therefore, the prospective parents' options are (a) to treat the embryo, (b) not to treat the embryo, and (c) to decide not to implant the embryo (Rulli, 2019), either choosing another embryo (if available) or giving up the attempt to pursue the pregnancy. Whereas the second option should be considered morally wrong, the third one should be morally permissible. Indeed, deciding not to implant Jeff-to-be does not affect any person because Jeff-to-be is not a person yet. Since no existing or future person is made worse off or better off by this choice, the third option should be considered a legitimate preference and, as a consequence, morally permissible. Therefore, there is no moral obligation to transfer Jeff-to-be.

Nonetheless, if reproducers decide to transfer into the uterus *that* specific embryo, then they face a moral obligation to treat the embryo first. By choosing to transfer a specific embryo, prospective parents are creating a particular individual with some interests not to be made worse off by the parents' choices. In other words, prospective parents are *recognizing* that embryo as their future child[25]. Hence, even though we are modifying an embryo that is not a person yet, we should treat it *as if* it were an actual person, in light of the expectation that that specific embryo will develop into a specific person. Due to the parents' act of recognizing the embryo as their future child, the designated *in vitro* embryo shares not only a biological continuity but also a *moral continuity* with the future person developed from such an embryo. In this way, the reproducers may justifiably be said to have some *parental* duty toward that embryo, a duty that falls within the sphere of procreative-parental responsibility.

Again, this does not entail any obligation to implant the modified embryo or to give birth to a child. Even if they had initially consented to the modification and implantation, they could "withdraw" their consent to having that specific child at any time by deciding either to abort or not to implant the modified embryo, or by selecting and transferring another embryo. However, if prospective parents are transferring a *specific* embryo, with the same condition as Jeff-to-be, in order to give birth to a numerically identical individual with such an embryo, then they are morally required to treat that embryo through rGE. Furthermore, this argument does not even require prospective parents to modify an embryo affected by a genetic disease rather than select another one, say Charlotte-to-be, not affected by that condition, if available. There is no moral consequences-based person-affecting reason to *prefer* genetic modification over selection.

To summarize, since the reasons that in Julia's case imply an obligation to treat her are also found in Jeff-to-be's case, we should accept a moral obligation to treat Jeff-to-be as well. In light of the availability of rGE techniques capable of preventing genetic diseases, prospective parents, *in some cases*, could be morally required to treat their future child, facing a greater moral obligation toward progeny than proposed by MTM. While in the context in which selective ARTs, including PGD, are the only available techniques, parents-to-be have no moral reasons related to the future child not to select an embryo free from disease X_1, in the context in which an rGE is available, safe, legal, and cheap, reproducers have a *prima facie* moral duty to treat the embryo affected by X_1 using Y_1. Therefore, while MTM is an effective instrument to guide reproductive choices when only genetic selection is available, it is not so when the additional option of rGE is present.

4.4 Redefining Procreative-Parental Responsibility in Light of Genome Editing

Since I have claimed that the availability of rGE commits one to accepting the Greater Moral Obligation View, I should explain what this implies in practice. It can be first argued that the availability of rGE generates moral obligations every time that prospective parents are about to transfer a specific human embryo that will develop into a person suffering from genetic diseases that meet the following criteria: (a) they are such diseases that are compatible with a life worth living, but they significantly impair the child's psychological and physical well-being and/or significantly curtail the reasonable range of opportunities for choosing their own life plan; (b) they are diseases for which, at the moment of IVF, safe treatment with rGE is available and legal, and it is not possible to treat them effectively *in vivo*[26] or after the birth of the child. Only under these circumstances can the child legitimately complain about the parents' decision, and this generates good reasons to limit the parents' procreative freedom.

Clarifications are needed for both criteria. Criterion (a) requires a further explanation regarding the concept of harm. In Chapter 3, I stated that the notion of harm, as discussed in the debate on the Non-Identity Problem, has a comparative and counterfactual nature and, in general terms, requires the existence of at least two scenarios in which a person P exists, with one scenario being worse for P than the other. However, this is not enough to state what conditions constitute harm since what it means to be disadvantaged or in a worse situation should be specified. In Julia and Jeff-to-be cases, I merely proposed conditions that intuitively seem to harm the persons involved. However, it should be recognized that we may encounter significant disagreement about which conditions specifically qualify as "worse" or which conditions are "worse" in morally relevant terms, thus giving rise to moral duties for someone to avoid them, especially given the varying degrees of severity these conditions may present. To avoid such disagreement and provide an account that many people can share, I limit my focus on conditions that can lead to disability, understood in terms compatible with both the welfarist and equal opportunities definitions of disability discussed in Chapter 2 (Sections 2.4.3 and 2.4.4). Although in some cases these definitions of what constitutes a harm are not exactly superimposable, there are nevertheless many situations where we can observe a convergence between them.

Criterion (b), instead, aims for neutrality regarding which technology or treatment to use to avoid conditions that meet criterion (a), if there is no evidence of greater effectiveness of one treatment compared to the other, and this choice does not cause negative consequences that were avoidable in the future person. Prescribing prospective parents to opt specifically for rGE when, *ceteris paribus*, effective options exist would be unnecessary and even irrational.

But these claims are still too general to be helpful. Therefore, it is crucial to specify the scenarios in which this obligation arises. In what follows, I propose two models or principles of procreative-parental responsibility that can guide future parents to assess *when* this new moral obligation toward offspring emerges in the procreative context.

4.4.1 The Bold Restriction of Procreative Autonomy

According to the Bold Restriction of Procreative Autonomy, prospective parents have a *prima facie* moral duty to procreate through IVF and then transfer into the uterus an embryo free from those genetic diseases that meet the aforementioned criteria (a) and (b). According to this proposal, every child born with such genetic diseases has a right to complain to their parents. Parents-to-be would have had the possibility to treat their child with rGE in order to avoid such genetic diseases. In reproduction through sexual intercourse, they have no control over the genetic traits of the created embryo: it would have no chance of being modified without the existence of a germinal manipulation technique directly in the mother's womb. Therefore, parents-to-be would have a moral duty to reproduce through IVF, allowing the future child to be treated with rGE. The Bold Restriction of Procreative Autonomy proposal would hence undermine the right to procreate through sexual intercourse.

Such a proposal is quite controversial, very demanding for reproducers, and – above all –hard to defend from a consequences-based person-affecting perspective.[27] In fact, the embryo created through sexual intercourse would never exist except as the result of sexual intercourse. Due to the specificity of human reproduction, the same embryo would not have existed *in vitro*, as a result of IVF, where parents could have treated it in order to avoid the genetic disease. The embryo E conceived through sexual intercourse is the result of the encounter between a sperm S and an oocyte O at a specific time. If prospective parents had decided to undergo IVF, there would have been an encounter between different gametes, say S_1 and O_1 at a different time, and accordingly, a different embryo, E_1 would have been implanted. Therefore, individuals conceived through sexual intercourse, having no possibility of being genetically modified, cannot complain to their parents because they could not have avoided a genetic disease that meets criteria (a) and (b). They could not have existed except under the conditions in which they also suffered from a genetic disease. The genetic inheritance they possess is the only one they could have had, as for the embryo selected through PGD. So, from a consequences-based person-affecting perspective, the right to traditional procreation is not undermined, despite the availability of rGE to treat genetic diseases that meet criteria (a) and (b). Prospective parents who want to procreate through sexual intercourse do not have a moral obligation to avoid the aforementioned genetic diseases in their progeny.

Advocates of Bold Restriction of Procreative Autonomy, however, might reply to this critique with the following argument: even though highly unlikely, it would not be impossible that the same sperm S could fertilize the same egg O both *in vitro* and during sexual intercourse, thereby producing the same embryo E. In this hypothetical perspective, it would not be wrong to claim that the embryo E conceived *in vivo*, from which the individual derived, could have been in a different place, that is, *in vitro*, where it could have been treated through rGE. Given this possibility, one might argue that the maternal womb does not constitute an ideal location for procreation and, therefore, faced with the emergence of genetic diseases that meet criteria (a) and (b), procreating naturally is morally problematic. By choosing to procreate naturally, the embryo is deprived of the possibility of being in the ideal place to undergo treatments to avoid genetic diseases that meet criteria (a) and (b).[28]

This counterobjection is quite controversial and seems to give excessive importance to statistically negligible probabilities, not considering the specificity of IVF: first, the person with a uterus intending to undergo IVF is administered drugs aimed at hyperovulation, namely, the induction of the development of a larger number of available egg cells than in the spontaneous cycle, in which usually only one egg cell becomes available. Therefore, reasonable doubts can be raised about whether, through the hyperovulation process, egg cell O can actually be used to produce embryo E. Moreover, ovarian stimulation could cause more oocytes to mature, but it could also even prevent the maturation of the specific egg O, also considering that to facilitate hyperovulation a drug can be used to suppress natural ovulation.

Second, even assuming that O is the egg cell used for creating the embryo that will then be implanted, or at least O is one of the egg cells produced and available for the artificial fertilization process, the chance of fertilization between O and the specific sperm S both *in vivo* and *in vitro* is infinitesimally small considering the number of sperms produced per ejaculation. In fact, the amount of sperm cells produced by each ejaculation ranges between 1.5 and 5 ml and depends on multiple factors, including the time between one ejaculation and the next one, and other individual factors. In addition, the number of sperms per ejaculation also varies, which is especially linked to the subject's health condition: this number varies from 200 to 500 million per ejaculation (Saladin, 2016).

Third, it is worth noting how slight time variations could influence the fertilization of the oocyte O by sperm S. Such data and considerations allow us to understand how drastically low, if not scientifically impossible, is the probability that the same pair of gametes' fertilization occurs *in vitro* and *in vivo*. Even if we acknowledge the existence of an infinitesimal possibility of such an event occurring, it would still be lower than other probabilities generally overlooked in moral calculus. If we considered the above reply valid, we would condemn ourselves to inaction because every action we take could potentially, however minimally, cause harm to someone. In light of this, the Bold Restriction of Procreative Autonomy must be rejected.

4.4.2   *The Mild Restriction of Procreative Autonomy*

A second and more reasonable proposal within the consequences-based person-affecting perspective is the Mild Restriction of Procreative Autonomy. According to this, prospective parents have a *prima facie* moral duty to transfer into the uterus an embryo without genetic diseases that meet criteria (a) and (b) only if they are already in the IVF process – that is, when *in vitro* embryos already exist – and if they want to have a child from one of those created embryos. In other words, given the availability of rGE, parents-to-be should not transfer the designated embryo unless the embryo has first been guaranteed to be free from genetic diseases that meet criteria (a) and (b). Only in such cases is it reasonable to speak of a person affecting harm and benefit, because the existing embryo that is designated to be transferred would have the possibility of being modified to avoid genetic diseases and disabilities. Clearly, this moral obligation is not toward the embryo, which is not a person yet, but toward the future person who will develop from that specific embryo.

Thus, procreative choices should be morally limited for reproducers who are already in the IVF process, which means that they are no longer morally entitled to transfer into the uterus any embryo with an expected life worth living, as allowed by MTM. Rather, parents-to-be are morally committed to transferring only those embryos that are free from genetic diseases that meet criteria (a) and (b), since if they transferred an embryo affected by these genetic diseases, the moral duty to use rGE before the transfer would emerge. Every person affected by a genetic disease who meets criteria (a) and (b) born thanks to IVF has the right to express complaints against their parents, since that person could have been treated with rGE and born without the genetic disease that harmed them. In practical terms, procreators act in a morally problematic way when (1) they transfer an embryo into the uterus after modifying it with rGE, causing a genetic disease that meets criterion (a); (2) they transfer one or more embryos with a disease that meets criteria (a) and (b) into the uterus without first treating them with rGE; and (3) they do not screen embryos to detect the presence of genetic diseases that meet criteria (a) and (b) and then transfer an embryo that will develop into a person with a genetic disease that meets those criteria.[29] In all three cases, it is possible to say that the future child is in a "harmed" condition that the parents could have avoided. Therefore, the child is entitled to express complaints toward their parents.

4.4.3 Procreative-Parental Responsibility and Other Non-Identity-Affecting Technologies

In the preceding sections, I primarily focused on rGE in early embryos. However, my argument also extends to other ARTs and prenatal treatments discussed in Chapter 1, some of which may become available in the future. A primary, straightforward point is that prospective parents who will employ *In Vitro* Gametogenesis (IVG) must grapple with the same obligations outlined earlier. This is because conceiving a child through IVG inevitably involves creating embryos *in vitro*, where there is the possibility to treat them via rGE. An IVG embryo, regardless of the cell from which it originates, shares the numerical identity with the future individual it will develop into. Consequently, prospective parents who decide to use IVG face a *prima facie* moral duty to transfer into the uterus an embryo without genetic diseases that meet criteria (a) and (b).

It is plausible to claim that some new obligations emerge also in light of the availability of Mitochondrial Replacement Therapy (MRT). Assessing such new moral obligations in this context is undoubtedly a complex topic and should be treated peculiarly in a separate setting. Here, I limit to claim that these duties would emerge only under certain circumstances, as MRT cannot always be considered a non-identity-affecting technique. As already mentioned in Chapter 1 (Subsection 1.1.6), MRT can occur in two different ways, namely, pronuclear transfer and maternal spindle transfer. Given their peculiarities, some might argue that the methodologies are not morally identical since the former replaces mitochondrial DNA in the embryo, while the latter replaces DNA in the oocyte. In light of this, some authors claim that while maternal spindle transfer affects the identity of the future individual and should be considered a "selective" practice, pronuclear transfer is a non-identity-affecting practice. Hence, the future individual might benefit or be harmed by the use or non-use of pronuclear transfer (Wrigley et al., 2015), and this would give rise to new moral obligations to resort to the reproductive technique under consideration in order to prevent the future individual from being affected by treatable mitochondrial diseases. As for rGE, this obligation would emerge only for prospective parents who have already begun the IVF process, which is a necessary step for MRT.

In addition, my argument applies to other techniques such as *in utero* gene therapy and fetal surgery. These are non-identity-affecting techniques for the same reasons mentioned above: a future child might be harmed or benefited by the act or omission of the parents-to-be and, hence, could potentially express legitimate complaints against them. Therefore, I argue that even in these cases, parents have a *prima facie* moral duty to treat embryos or fetuses with diseases or conditions that meet the aforementioned criterion (a) and a revised version of criterion (b), namely, (b*): conditions for which a safe and effective treatment has been discovered at the time of pregnancy using the techniques mentioned above, and it is not possible to treat them more or at least equally effectively after the child's birth. Notice that the moral obligation to resort to such treatments would be directed not only to procreators already in the IVF process but to *all* prospective parents. This generates a moral obligation to resort to prenatal genetic tests to assess the presence of any diseases that meet criteria (a) and (b*). Therefore, there is an even greater extension of procreative responsibility toward offspring in the sense that it concerns many more procreators.[30] As in the rGE context, if the fetus is not yet considered a person, the pregnant person or the couple could decide to terminate the pregnancy.

However, we should keep in mind that *in utero* genetic modifications or fetal therapy certainly imply more significant physical and psychological burdens than the context in which Mild Restriction of Procreative Autonomy applies, namely, after the parent has undergone IVF. They imply invasive interventions on the pregnant person's body, who might feel morally obliged to take disproportionate risks to treat the embryo or fetus. Hence, such considerations should be carefully balanced, emphasizing that the moral obligations discussed in this chapter are *prima facie* and not absolute.

Finally, let us consider the possibility of ectogenesis in both its partial and complete forms. The potential advantage of ectogenesis would be to allow the embryo or fetus to develop, partially or completely, in an environment not affected by possible illnesses of the mother, alcohol or drugs that the pregnant person could use, and, more importantly, being treated through fetal therapy or genetic treatment to avoid disability or diseases. At first glance, I acknowledge that ectogenesis cannot be directly described as a non-identity-affecting technique, since this is simply a way of gestation that does not *by itself* affect the future individual.[31] However, I consider it a non-identity-affecting technique because it would make it possible to have the ideal place to apply interventions – such as genetic modification (germline and somatic) and fetal therapy – on the embryo and fetus during development in a more secure way than in the uterus.

With this in mind, I consider ectogenesis in its most far and hypothetical form, namely, the total or complete one. In this context, the moral scenario would be quite similar to that discussed with regard to rGE: there may be a *prima facie* moral duty to resort to ectogenesis only for prospective parents who are already in the IVF process in order to avoid conditions that meet the criteria discussed above. If I consider the possibility of a partial ectogenesis that allows the viability of a partially developed embryo or fetus several weeks before birth outside the mother's womb, then moral reasons would emerge to transfer the fetus into the artificial womb for as long as possible to guarantee the future child any treatments that meet the aforementioned criteria. Clearly, this kind of partial ectogenesis would make prenatal treatments easier and safer, in particular for the pregnant person. However, other psychological and physical burdens on the pregnant person who would have to undergo surgery to remove the fetus from the uterus at a certain stage of pregnancy must be carefully considered and balanced against the moral reasons I have presented here.

To sum up, although each of the discussed non-identity-affecting techniques certainly deserves a more in-depth reflection, there are good reasons to extend the Greater Moral Obligation View also to them, arguing that the development of them expands procreative-parental responsibility and, consequently, procreative responsibility. Even stemming from the minimum requirements of consequences-based person-affecting morality here assumed, prospective parents will have greater moral obligations toward offspring once such techniques are made available, safe, legal, and cheap.

4.5   Integrating Procreative-Parental Responsibility with Reproductive Responsibility

As I argued, the Mild Restriction of Procreative Autonomy can be described as a procreative-parental responsibility model. While this book primarily addresses procreative-parental responsibilities, it is important to note that the procreative responsibility sphere encompasses more than just the obligations future parents have toward their children. Reproductive choices not only affect offspring but can also have morally significant implications for other children, family members, and, more generally, others. Although many people agree that parents have special obligations to their own children, it is also true that overly favoring one's offspring to the detriment of others – for instance, through nepotism practices – is still morally problematic. Therefore, it is plausible that, in the reproductive context, there are moral constraints that go beyond the interests of the future child and that these must be integrated with considerations concerning procreative-parental responsibility.

For this reason, some models of *reproductive* responsibility have been proposed, discussing the moral duties that reproducers have toward third parties. Note I do not aim to offer an exhaustive reflection on reproductive responsibility issues, but I have a more modest purpose: recognizing that the moral duties arising in the procreative-parental context must be considered together with other obligations that might emerge in light of considerations that go beyond the concerns toward the future child. In other words, below I provide some considerations intending to integrate them with the procreative-parental responsibility models discussed in previous sections. Integrating these two distinct categories of procreative obligations is a necessary step to formalize a comprehensive procreative responsibility model, namely, one that considers all the various morally relevant reasons involved in the decision to procreate a new child.

Reproductive responsibility models can be either impersonal or person-affecting in nature. In Subsection 3.3.1, I argued that PPB should be considered a reproductive responsibility model. If we fully embrace its premises, it seems reasonable to say that PPB should not only be focused on the well-being of the future child but adopt a more general interpretation aimed at maximizing the aggregate well-being in the world. Nonetheless, the Principle of Procreative (or, more properly, Reproductive) Beneficence remains an impersonal model even in its generalized sense. Nevertheless, other reproductive responsibility models only embrace a consequences-based person-affecting morality. According to these models, reproductive choices hold moral significance only as long as they have effects on already actual people.

One of the most discussed reproductive responsibility models is Procreative Altruism, proposed by Thomas Douglas and Katrien Devolder.

Henceforth, I will refer to it as Reproductive Altruism, which aligns with the terminology proposed in Chapter 2. According to this model:

> If couples (or single reproducers) have decided to have a child, and selection is possible, they have significant moral reason to select a child whose existence can be expected to contribute more to (or detract less from) the well-being of others than any alternative child they could have.
>
> (Douglas & Devolder, 2013, p. 403)

Generally, some traits considered advantageous for the individual may have indirect positive consequences for society. For instance, intelligence, empathy, and creativity might contribute not only to the well-being or flourishing of the individual possessing them but also to society at large, and hence, they may be regarded as a "public good" (Anomaly, 2014). On the contrary, some characteristics might be advantageous for an individual but disadvantageous for many others. Let us assume the discovery of a gene combination that makes carriers more inclined than average to breach socially advantageous cooperation norms to pursue personal interests. While it may be beneficial for the carrier to possess this gene combination, this is not the case for society (Douglas & Devolder, 2013).

Furthermore, whereas it might be better for society if more individuals with the O-negative blood type were born (serving as universal donors), from an individual perspective, it would be better to have the AB-positive blood type, making one a universal recipient (Elster, 2011). Reproductive Altruism highlights significant moral reasons, or *prima facie* moral duties, to generate individuals through ARTs with traits that benefit existing individuals, even if these traits would not necessarily benefit the future individual. According to Douglas and Devolder, Reproductive Altruism prescriptions should be considered in conjunction with procreative-parental considerations to provide a better practical tool for informing procreative choices.

Reproductive Altruism is similar to another model, namely, the Generalized Procreative Non-Maleficence (henceforth Generalized Reproductive Non-Maleficence) proposed by Ben Saunders, although the latter seems to demand less from reproducers than the former. According to this model:

> Prospective parents should consider the interests of others, rather than only the child, but [...] they need only avoid harm to others, rather than being required to produce the greatest possible benefit.
>
> (Saunders, 2017, p. 554)

The Generalized Reproductive Non-Maleficence model is not as maximizing as the previous one. It embrace the moral intuition that our duties to others are limited and that people have stronger moral reasons not to harm others, compared to benefiting them (Saunders, 2017). However, in agreement with Devolder and Douglas, accepting this does not mean that benefiting someone is morally irrelevant. The authors argue that Reproductive Altruism does not necessarily commit to maximization, even *pro tanto*, of benefits through the reproductive act, while still considering it morally significant to benefit third parties (Douglas & Devolder, 2013). My aim here is not to discuss which of the two models is more appropriate; I just observe the emergence of reproductive moral duties that are not only related to the procreative-parental sphere. Regardless of their level of demandingness, the request of the two models largely overlaps since they require considering the interests of third parties and not just the interests of the future individual in the procreative choice, from a non-necessarily maximizing perspective.

These models have different implications depending on the ARTs considered. In the selective context, they should be integrated with MTM: since MTM does not offer moral reasons to select an individual with certain characteristics over another, provided they have a life worth living, reproductive responsibility considerations or requests would not conflict with the interest of the future individual, but only with the preferences of the parents-to-be and their reproductive autonomy. Thus, as Roberts argues, it is possible to consider genetic selection a practice able to generate person-affecting harms or benefits if one believes that a person's birth can generally worsen or ameliorate the lives of actual, existing people (Roberts, 2009). In light of this, reproductive responsibility considerations would take on at least significant weight, despite not being definitive, in the reproductive choice. In this context, procreators would have a moral duty to avoid selecting a child with traits that could cause burdens or costs at the family and social level, such as certain severe genetic diseases (Douglas & Devolder, 2013) and, assuming it becomes possible in the future, certain character traits.

Recently, it was suggested that these models are not sufficient to grasp all reproductive responsibility prescriptions because they fail to detect certain eminent justice-related issues that may arise. Herjeet Kaur Marway proposes the Principle of Procreative Justice, which we should rename the Principle of Reproductive Justice. She invites us to imagine a scenario where Bo, after undergoing IVF, has the choice to transfer into the uterus either embryo A, likely to develop a lighter skin tone, or embryo B, likely to develop a darker skin tone. She claims that reproducers have strong *pro tanto* moral reasons to avoid perpetuating race or color injustice in their selection decision (Marway, 2023). Therefore, in this case, Bo would have some reasons to avoid choosing embryo A. According to the author, both Reproductive Altruism and Generalized Reproductive Non-Maleficence could provide reasons not to select embryo A. For example, selecting for dark skin serves to mitigate the "expressive" harms inflicted on darker-skinned groups or counteracts the "eugenic" harms that occur with a reduction in darker-skinned people via lighter skin selection. However, according to Marway, these reasons would be mostly speculative and would not capture the genuine justice-based reasons that should be considered. It is not my intention to evaluate the plausibility of this proposal – which I believe applies, for instance, to the case of sex selection (Hendl, 2017) – but to highlight how reproductive responsibility may involve not only reasons of beneficence and non-maleficence but also of justice.

Applying reproductive responsibility models is more complex when we consider the availability of non-identity-affecting techniques, such as rGE, *in utero* gene therapy, and fetal therapy. As I argued in previous sections, in these contexts, there is the possibility of harming or benefiting the future individual, potentially triggering a conflict of interests. But here we should acknowledge that generally benefiting an individual, for instance, by preventing severe genetic diseases, coincides with promoting the welfare of society. In most cases of using non-identity-affecting techniques, there would be moral reasons not only related to the individual's well-being or interests but also arising from the well-being of other actual people. However, in cases where a conflict still emerges, the combined application of procreative-parental responsibility models with reproductive responsibility models could be more complex.

Some might argue that considering social interest in procreative choices could lead to a scenario where the interests of future children are systematically frustrated in favor of societal well-being. This would be true if one adopted a very demanding maximizing view of reproductive responsibility but, as argued above, none of the presented models is committed to this problematic assumption. Indeed, although reproductive responsibility may take on primary importance in selective contexts (Saunders, 2017), one can reasonably argue that, in relation to non-identity-affecting practices, reproductive responsibility models are compatible with considering the interests of the child as lexically prior to those of society (Douglas & Devolder, 2013, p. 414). In light of this, one could reasonably argue that the Mild Restriction of Procreative Autonomy requests in the rGE context should have priority over those required by reproductive responsibility models. This would be consistent with our considered moral views on parenthood, whereby parents have special duties toward their offspring.

However, even accepting such a lexical priority, there might be cases where societal interests could outweigh the future child's interest. Such scenarios could occur if the future child had a trait potentially harmful to others, and its elimination through rGE treatment did not significantly compromise the individual's physical and mental well-being or did not reduce their access to a reasonable range of different life plans. Considering, for example, a genetic combination that makes carriers more inclined than average to violate socially advantageous cooperation norms, it seems reasonable to argue that prospective parents have some *prima facie* moral duty to avoid benefiting the future individual at the expense of significantly harming the well-being of others, since eliminating such a trait does not appear to significantly disadvantage the future individual. Consider another scenario in which society's interest might be paramount: the potential genetic enhancement of future individuals. In such a context, treating fetuses or embryos to ensure they receive positional goods – when not everyone is enhanced or has access to such enhancement – could be ethically challenging. These treatments could raise justice issues concerning potential fairness distortions stemming from advantages bestowed upon individuals through certain enhancement interventions (Buchanan et al., 2000). Such concerns prompted the Nuffield Council (2018) to claim that rGE may be acceptable as long as it cannot reasonably be expected to create or exacerbate social divisions or lead to the unchecked marginalization or disadvantage of particular societal groups. While this duty primarily pertains to society as a whole, it might also hold relevance for prospective parents.

Finally, it is important to recall that reproductive responsibility can be not only *quality-oriented* but also *quantity-oriented*. This does not pertain to decisions about which child to procreate or the treatment that should be ensured for the future child. Instead, it concerns decisions regarding whether to bring children into existence and how many children to have. As detailed in Chapter 2 (Subsection 2.3.2), these considerations are especially pertinent in scenarios of overpopulation and underpopulation, though they are not confined to these contexts. In this discussion, the possible moral conflict is between the aspirations of parents-would-be and the interests of existing third parties. A quantity-based reproductive responsibility model may contend that prospective parents should have no more than one child per couple[32]. However, some authors consider such an obligation quite supererogatory and untenable (Overall, 2012): Trevor Hedberg proposes instead that parents-would-be should ideally consider having no more than one child each reproduces – hence, two baby per couple – particularly if they reside in countries with significant ecological footprints per capita (Hedberg, 2021)[33]. Here, I leave open the question about how many children a responsible reproducer should have because more discussion is needed.

Notes

1 Subsection 4.2.2, Section 4.3, Subsections 4.3.1 and 4.3.2 discuss concepts already presented in Battisti (2021), frequently employing the same wording as the original published article.

2 Notice that I do not use *if and only if* but *only if*, since I do not want to commit myself to consider every harm, here considered as a decrease of well-being or opportunities, morally wrong, and every benefit, namely, an increase of well-being, morally good.

3 Generally, person-affecting morality is associated with the so-called moral actualism, according to which only actual people morally count (Hare, 2007). Although this thesis is particularly intuitive, it has been criticized by Roberts, who argues that the person-affecting approach can be combined with non-actualist perspectives according to which even merely possible persons are morally relevant (Roberts, 2011b).

4 Among the major supporters of a person-affecting approach to the Non-Identity Problem are Narveson (1973), Schwartz (1978, 1979), Heyd (1988, 1992); Roberts (1998), Magni (2019, 2020, 2021), Bennett (2009, 2014), and Boonin (2014, 2020).

5 Roberts' position becomes significantly more complex when dealing with other non-identity cases unrelated to Anna and Eddie's case. In line with Matthew Hanser (1990, 2009), Roberts morally distinguishes cases like Anna's from cases like the Risky Policy. The latter, in fact, would not be cases of non-identity, as, unlikely as it may be, it would not be impossible for the same individual existing under policy A to have also existed under policy B. The non-identity of the risky policy is thus a matter of probability (Roberts, 2007). This reasoning does not apply to the cases at hand, in which an individual cannot exist unless affected by a specific genetic disease. In this section, I have considered the argument solely in reference to this last category of non-identity cases, which includes the procreative choices under examination here.

6 Nevertheless, we can acknowledge that in some contexts, we have obligations toward people who do not yet exist and whose identity is not defined at the time of the action or omission under moral scrutiny. Consider the case of an individual hiding a bomb in a city that will explode in 200 years, killing hundreds of thousands. Since this action will not affect the identities of people who will exist in 200 years and who the bomb will kill, it seems plausible to argue that the terrorist's action is still bound by the interests of actual people.

7 Note that in this context, I use "intelligence" and "IQ" interchangeably. However, while IQ tests are typically seen as measures of specific types of intelligence, they may not adequately encompass broader facets of human intelligence, like creativity and social insight.

8 The idea that greater intelligence does not promote well-being was discussed by Carter and Gordon (2013), while the opposing thesis can be found in Saunders (2015).

9 For a similar formulation, see Buller & Bauer (2011). This model is also known as the Principle of Procreative Non-Maleficence, which was recently proposed by van der Hout et al. (2019). Notice that another Principle of Procreative Non-Maleficence has been proposed by Baldwin. He argues that not only should parents not bring into life those not worthy of living but also that, if one were to use IVF and PGD, it would be morally obligatory to create lives better than what an individual born without such selective procedures would have had (Baldwin, 2014). Nonetheless, I believe that the latter model cannot be justified from a person-affecting perspective, since it is not possible to make the comparison proposed by the author between the life of the person born after PGD and the life of the person who could have been born without the use of this technique.

10 As argued in Chapter 2, I am aware that defining deafness as a disability is controversial, and this issue for many remains open. I have chosen to mention it since the selection of embryos with deafness through PGD is one of the

concrete examples of the use of selective techniques not to avoid genetic diseases, but aimed at seeking specific traits that many consider disabling. In this regard, for a contribution on this topic, see Wallis (2020).

11 Note that Piller accepts the existence/non-existence comparability only from the moment in which one exists since he considers the concept of "benefitting" a relationship between a person P and an event E that benefits P (Piller, 2023).

12 Feinberg follows a similar strategy in Feinberg (1986).

13 For a discussion on the Asymmetry, see McMahan (1981, 2009).

14 For a discussion, see McMahan (2009).

15 Roberts suggests a different solution but still compatible with my conclusion. Starting from a person-affecting comparativist approach, Roberts embraces a "variabilist" perspective, which holds that all people, both actual and merely possible, should be considered morally; nonetheless, their loss (e.g., having been born with a life not worth living, not having been born with a life worth living) is morally relevant depending on the position in which the individual finds themselves (Roberts, 2011b). In other words, the loss of actual persons would be significant, unlike that of merely possible persons.

16 In this book, I do not consider the timing of the embryo transfer to the uterus as a relevant factor in guiding procreative decisions in the context of IVF. However, there may be person-affecting reasons for delaying the transfer of one or more already created embryos into the uterus thanks to embryo cryopreservation. This decision could be based on the reasonable expectation that the future economic, social, and emotional context for the child would be more favorable than if the prospective parents proceeded with the transfer immediately. Therefore, a new type of person-affecting harm and benefit would emerge, which I call "repro-timing harm and benefit". This concept will be further explored in my forthcoming works, Battisti (forthcoming a, forthcoming b).

17 Since in Chapter 1 I assumed that the procedure is safe, I do not consider the possibility that the PGD process might damage the embryo, resulting in adverse consequences for the person who will develop from such an embryo.

18 I presented the concept of numerical identity in Chapter 3 (Section 3.2). Notice that this assumption is controversial: I discuss objections and defend this assumption in Chapter 5 (Section 5.1).

19 In this work, I consciously refrain from describing rGE as a form of "therapy". While rGE could be considered therapeutic, perhaps to a greater extent than PGD (Cavaliere, 2018), this designation remains highly controversial. For further discussion on this topic, see Rulli (2019) and Palacios-González (2021).

20 I owe this suggestion to Sergio Filippo Magni.

21 This bizarre but fascinating case is reported by Douglas and Devolder (2022).

22 For a discussion on the concept of "complaint" in the context of genetic engineering, see Delaney (2011).

23 We should notice that Julia's case and Jeff-to-be's case are not perfectly equivalent, morally speaking, and this could raise problems for the claim just made. Indeed, we encounter further elements in Julia's case because we also need to take into account the current child's suffering, whereas this is not the case for Jeff-to-be. However, all else being equal, Julia's case seems to entail a moral obligation to treat for reasons that also apply in Jeff-to-be's case. In fact, both Julia and Jeff could experience harm from the parents' decision to avoid treatment, and this stands as a strong reason to favor a moral duty to care, independent from Julia's current suffering.

24 Here I assume that Julia is already a person. Although this assumption is supported by common sense morality, it is controversial (Giubilini & Minerva,
2013; Tooley, 1985).

25 For a position that aligns with such analysis, which is provided in the context
of prenatal harm occurring during pregnancy, see Howard (2023).

26 I am referring to fetal therapy and *in utero* gene therapy. For a discussion about
responsibility in the context of fetal therapy, see Kanaris (2017).

27 In Chapter 7, I will argue that the model of Bold Restriction of Procreative
Autonomy can be partially rehabilitated by considering the moral relevance of
the intentions and attitudes of the prospective parents.

28 I believe that this defense is in line with Roberts' argument briefly mentioned
above, according to which some definite cases of non-identity are instead cases
of probability (Roberts, 2007). Roberts' argument presents the same problems
as the model of procreative responsibility under consideration since, as will be
seen below, it seems to give excessive importance to infinitesimal probabilities.
For a critique of Roberts that uses a similar argument, see Greene (2016).

29 Notice that this argument mainly applies when and if it becomes possible to
first screen embryos genetically and then safely and effectively modify any embryos affected by genetic diseases. As previously stated in Chapter 1 (Subsection 1.2.1.1), this possibility faces technical challenges, especially concerning
the early applications of rGE, because experts believe genome editing, to avoid
mosaicism risks, should occur before the first cell division. However, conduct-
ing genetic tests on embryos like PGD at this stage would mean destroying the
embryo. In the future, scientific advancements in genome editing techniques
and preimplantation genetic tests could overcome these challenges. According
to Hershlag and Bristow, such progress seems desirable if we aim to implement
rGE in human reproduction. For a detailed discussion on this, see Hershlag and
Bristow (2018).

30 This obligation seems to some extent also accepted on an intuitive level, if we
consider that parents who subject the fetus to fetal therapy for spina bifida justify their choice mainly by appealing to parental responsibility (Crombag et al.,
2021).

31 Here, I am not considering any epigenetic changes that might emerge from the
difference in place of gestation.

32 This position has been maintained, among others, by Conly (2016), who even
argues in favor of legal, and not just moral, restrictions on reproduction.

33 A similar position has been endorsed also by Overall (2012).

References

Alonso, M., & Savulescu, J. (2021). He Jiankui´s gene-editing experiment and the
non-identity problem. *Bioethics*, *35*(6), 563–573.

Anomaly, J. (2014). Public goods and procreation. *Monash Bioethics Review*,
32(3–4), 172–188.

Arrhenius, G. (2000). *Future Generations – A challenge for moral theory*. Uppsala
University Press.

Baldwin, T. (2014). Choosing who: What is wrong with making better children? In
J. R. Spencer & A. du Bois-Pedain (Eds.), *Freedom and responsibility in reproductive choice*. Hart Publishing.

Battisti, D. (2021). Affecting future individuals: Why and when germline genome editing entails a greater moral obligation towards progeny. *Bioethics*, 35(5), 487–495.

Battisti, D. (2023). Attitudes, intentions and procreative responsibility in current and future assisted reproduction. *Bioethics*, 37(5), 449–461.

Battisti, D. (forthcoming a). Il danno prenatale temporale. *Paradigmi*: special issue "Etica e Generazione".

Battisti, D. (forthcoming b). Repro-Timing Harm and Benefit in Assisted Reproduction: Person-Affecting Reasons Before the Advent of Genome Editing. *American Journal of Bioethics: AJOB*.

Bennett, R. (2009). The fallacy of the Principle of Procreative Beneficence. *Bioethics*, 23(5), 265–273.

Bennett, R. (2014). When intuition is not enough. Why the Principle of Procreative Beneficence must work much harder to justify its eugenic vision. *Bioethics*, 28(9), 447–455.

Boonin, D. (2008). How to solve the non-identity problem. *Public Affairs Quarterly*, 22(2), 129–159.

Boonin, D. (2014). *Non-identity problem and the ethics of future people*. Oxford University Press.

Boonin, D. (2020). Solving the non-identity problem: A reply to Gardner, Kumar, Malek, Mulgan, Roberts and Wasserman. *Law Ethics and Philosophy*, 127–156.

Bradley, B. (2013). Asymmetries in benefiting, harming and creating. *The Journal of Ethics*, 17(1–2), 37–49.

Buchanan, A., Brock, D. W., Daniels, N., & Wikler, D. (2000). *From chance to choice*. Cambridge University Press.

Buller, T., & Bauer, S. (2011). Balancing procreative autonomy and parental responsibility. *Cambridge Quarterly of Healthcare Ethics: CQ: The International Journal of Healthcare Ethics Committees*, 20(2), 268–276.

Carter, J. A., & Gordon, E. C. (2013). Intelligence, wellbeing and procreative beneficence. *Journal of Applied Philosophy*, 30(2), 122–135.

Cavaliere, G. (2018). Genome editing and assisted reproduction: Curing embryos, society or prospective parents? *Medicine, Health Care, and Philosophy*, 21(2), 215–225.

Conly, S. (2016). *One child: Do we have a right to more?*. Oxford University Press.

Crombag, N., Sacco, A., Stocks, B., De Vloo, P., van der Merwe, J., Gallagher, K., David, A., Marlow, N., & Deprest, J. (2021). 'We did everything we could'- a qualitative study exploring the acceptability of maternal-fetal surgery for spina bifida to parents. *Prenatal Diagnosis*, 41(8), 910–921.

DeGrazia, D. (2016). *Procreative responsibility in view of what parents owe their children* (L. Francis, Ed.). Oxford University Press.

Delaney, J. J. (2011). Possible people, complaints, and the distinction between genetic planning and genetic engineering. *Journal of Medical Ethics*, 37(7), 410–414.

Douglas, T., & Devolder, K. (2013). Procreative altruism: Beyond individualism in reproductive selection. *The Journal of Medicine and Philosophy*, 38(4), 400–419.

Douglas, T., & Devolder, K. (2022). Gene editing, identity and benefit. *The Philosophical Quarterly*, 72(2), 305–325.

Elster, J. (2011). Procreative beneficence: Cui bono? *Bioethics, 25*(9), 482–488.

Feeney, O., & Rakić, V. (2021). Genome editing and 'disenhancement': Considerations on issues of non-identity and genetic pluralism. *Humanities and Social Sciences Communications, 8*(1). https://doi.org/10.1057/s41599-021-00795-w

Feinberg, J. (1986). Wrongful life and the counterfactual element in harming. *Social Philosophy and Policy, 4*(1), 145–178.

Feit, N. (2016). Comparative harm, creation and death. *Utilitas, 28*(2), 136–163.

Gavaghan, C. (2007). *Defending the genetic supermarket: Law and ethics of selecting the next generation.* Routledge-Cavendish.

Giubilini, A., & Minerva, F. (2013). After-birth abortion: Why should the baby live? *Journal of Medical Ethics, 39*(5), 261–263.

Glover, J. (2006). *Choosing children.* Oxford University Press.

Greene, M. E. (2016). Roberts on depletion: How much better can we do for future people? *Utilitas, 28*(1), 108–118.

Hanser, M. (1990). Harming future people. *Philosophy & Public Affairs, 19*(1), 47–70.

Hanser, M. (2009). Harming and Procreating. In M. A. Roberts & D. T. Wasserman (Eds.), *Harming future persons* (pp. 179–199). Springer Netherlands.

Hare, C. (2007). Voices from another world: Must we respect the interests of people who do not, and will never, exist? *Ethics, 117*(3), 498–523.

Hedberg, T. (2021). *The environmental impact of overpopulation.* Routledge.

Hendl, T. (2017). A feminist critique of justifications for sex selection. *Journal of Bioethical Inquiry, 14*(3), 427–438.

Herissone-Kelly, P. (2012). Wrongs, preferences, and the selection of children: A critique of Rebecca Bennett's argument against the principle of procreative beneficence. *Bioethics, 26*(8), 447–454.

Hershlag, A., & Bristow, S. L. (2018). Editing the human genome: Where ART and science intersect. *Journal of Assisted Reproduction and Genetics, 35*(8), 1367–1370.

Heyd, D. (1988). Procreation and value can ethics deal with futurity problems? *Philosophia (Ramat-Gan, Israel), 18*(2–3), 151–170.

Heyd, D. (1992). *Genethics.* University of California Press.

Howard, N. R. (2023). Maternal autonomy and prenatal harm. *Bioethics, 37*(3), 246–255.

Kanaris, C. (2017). Foetal surgery and using in utero therapies to reduce the degree of disability after birth. Could it be morally defensible or even morally required? *Medicine, Health Care, and Philosophy, 20*(1), 131–146.

Magni, S. F. (2019). Procreative beneficence toward whom? *Croatian Journal of Philosophy, 19*(1), 71–80.

Magni, S. F. (2020). Person-affecting procreative beneficence. *Phenomenology and Mind, 19*, 124.

Magni, S. F. (2021). In defence of person-affecting procreative beneficence. *Bioethics, 35*(5), 473–479.

Marway, H. K. (2023). Procreative justice and genetic selection for skin colour. *Bioethics, 37*(4), 389–398.

McMahan, J. (1981). Problems of population choice. *Ethics, 92*(1), 97–127.

McMahan, J. (1994). Review of David Heyd, genethics: Moral issues in the creation of people. *The Philosophical Review*, 103(3), 557.

McMahan, J. (2009). Asymmetries in the morality of causing people to exist. In M. A. Roberts & D. T. Wasserman (Eds.), *Harming future persons* (pp. 49–68). Springer Netherlands.

McMahan, J., & Savulescu, J. (2023). Reasons and reproduction: Gene editing and genetic selection. *The American Journal of Bioethics: AJOB*, 1–11. https://doi.org/10.1080/15265161.2023.2250288.

Narveson, J. (1973). Moral problems of population. *The Monist*, 57(1), 62–86.

Nuffield's Council. (2018). *Genome editing and human reproduction: Social and ethical issues.*

Omerbasic, A. (2018). Genome editing, non-identity and the notion of harm. In M. Braun, H. Schickl, & P. Dabrock (Eds.), *Between Moral Hazard and legal uncertainty* (pp. 67–81). Springer Fachmedien Wiesbaden.

Overall, C. (2012). *Why have children?* MIT Press.

Palacios-González, C. (2021). Reproductive genome editing interventions are therapeutic, sometimes. *Bioethics*, 35(6), 557–562.

Parfit, D. (1982). Future generations: Further problems. *Philosophy & Public Affairs*, 11(2), 113–172.

Parfit, D. (1984). *Reasons and persons.* Oxford University Press.

Persson, I. (2009). Rights and the asymmetry between creating good and bad lives. In *Harming future persons* (pp. 29–47). Springer Netherlands.

Petersen, T. S. (2001). Generocentrism: A critical discussion of David Heyd. *Philosophia (Ramat-Gan, Israel)*, 28(1–4), 411–423.

Piller, C. (2023). Glad to be alive: How we can compare a person's existence and her non-existence in terms of what is better or worse for this person. *Analytic Philosophy.* https://doi.org/10.1111/phib.12302

Ranisch, R. (2020). Germline genome editing versus preimplantation genetic diagnosis: Is there a case in favour of germline interventions? *Bioethics*, 34(1), 60–69.

Ranisch, R. (2022). Procreative Beneficence and Genome Editing. *The American Journal of Bioethics: AJOB*, 22(9), 20–22.

Roberts, M. A. (1998). *Child versus childmaker.* Rowman & Littlefield.

Roberts, M. A. (2003). Can it ever be better never to have existed at all? Person-based consequentialism and a new repugnant conclusion. *Journal of Applied Philosophy*, 20(2), 159–185.

Roberts, M. A. (2007). The non-identity fallacy: Harm, probability and another look at Parfit's depletion example. *Utilitas*, 19(3), 267–311.

Roberts, M. A. (2009). The nonidentity problem and the two envelope problem: When is one act better for a person than another? In M. A. Roberts & D. T. Wasserman (Eds.), *Harming future persons* (pp. 201–228). Springer Netherlands.

Roberts, M. A. (2011a). An asymmetry in the ethics of procreation. *Philosophy Compass*, 6(11), 765–776.

Roberts, M. A. (2011b). The asymmetry: A solution. *Theoria*, 77(4), 333–367.

Robertson, J. A. (1994). *Children of choice: Freedom and the new reproductive technologies.* Princeton University Press.

Rulli, T. (2019). Reproductive CRISPR does not cure disease. *Bioethics*, *33*(9), 1072–1082.

Saladin, K. S. (2016). *Human anatomy* (5th ed.). McGraw-Hill Education.

Saunders, B. (2015). Procreative beneficence, intelligence, and the optimization problem. *The Journal of Medicine and Philosophy*, *40*(6), 653–668.

Saunders, B. (2017). First, do no harm: Generalized procreative non-maleficence. *Bioethics*, *31*(7), 552–558.

Savulescu, J., & Alonso, M. (2022). Is gene editing harmless? Two arguments for gene editing. *The American Journal of Bioethics: AJOB*, *22*(9), 23–28.

Savulescu, J., & Kahane, G. (2016). *Understanding procreative beneficence* (L. Francis, Ed.). Oxford University Press.

Schaefer, G. O. (2020). Can reproductive genetic manipulation save lives? *Medicine, Health Care, and Philosophy*, *23*(3), 381–386.

Schwartz, T. (1978). Obligations to posterity. In R. Sikora & B. Barry (Eds.), *Obligations to future generations* (pp. 3–13). Temple University Press.

Schwartz, T. (1979). Welfare judgments and future generations. *Theory and Decision*, *11*, 181–194.

Singer, P. (1993). Review of David Heyd genethics: Moral issues in the creation of people. *Bioethics*, *7*(1), 63–67.

Singer, P. (2015). *Practical ethics* (2nd ed.). Cambridge University Press (Virtual Publishing).

Sparrow, R. (2022). Human germline genome editing: On the nature of our reasons to genome edit. *The American Journal of Bioethics: AJOB*, *22*(9), 4–15.

Sprigge, T. L. S. (1968). I. Professor Narveson's utilitarianism. *Inquiry (Oslo, Norway)*, *11*(1–4), 332–346.

Stramondo, J. (2017). Disabled by design: Justifying and limiting parental authority to choose future children with pre-implantation genetic diagnosis. *Kennedy Institute of Ethics Journal*, *27*(4), 475–500.

Tooley, M. (1985). *Abortion and infanticide*. Oxford University Press.

van der Hout, S., Dondorp, W., & de Wert, G. (2019). The aims of expanded universal carrier screening: Autonomy, prevention, and responsible parenthood. *Bioethics*, *33*(5), 568–576.

Vollset, S. E., Goren, E., Yuan, C.-W., Cao, J., Smith, A. E., Hsiao, T., Bisignano, C., Azhar, G. S., Castro, E., Chalek, J., Dolgert, A. J., Frank, T., Fukutaki, K., Hay, S. I., Lozano, R., Mokdad, A. H., Nandakumar, V., Pierce, M., Pletcher, M., ... Murray, C. J. L. (2020). Fertility, mortality, migration, and population scenarios for 195 countries and territories from 2017 to 2100: A forecasting analysis for the Global Burden of Disease Study. *Lancet*, *396*(10258), 1285–1306.

Wallis, J. M. (2020). Is it ever morally permissible to select for deafness in one's child? *Medicine, Health Care, and Philosophy*, *23*(1), 3–15.

Weinberg, R. (2013). Existence: Who needs it? The non-identity problem and merely possible people. *Bioethics*, *27*(9), 471–484.

Wrigley, A., Wilkinson, S., & Appleby, J. B. (2015). Mitochondrial replacement: Ethics and identity. *Bioethics*, *29*(9), 631–638.

5 Is Genome Editing Really Non-Identity-Affecting? A Defense of the Greater Moral Obligation View

The central thesis proposed in the previous chapter is that the availability of reproductive Genome Editing (rGE) commits us to accept a greater moral obligation toward progeny than those implied by the Minimal Threshold Model (MTM) where only genetic selection is possible. I called this position the Greater Moral Obligation View. From a consequences-based person-affecting perspective, it implies the Mild Restriction of Procreative Autonomy, according to which prospective parents have a greater moral obligation toward progeny only if they are within the *In Vitro* Fertilization (IVF) process. In the final chapter of this book, I will try to argue that the Greater Moral Obligation View gives us reasons to accept the Bold Restriction of Procreative Autonomy, if we consider the moral relevance of intentions and attitudes in a way compatible with person-affecting morality. However, here we should notice that in any case, the Greater Moral Obligation View rests on the assumption that rGE is a non-identity-affecting practice, namely, a procedure that will affect a person who will surely exist, harming or benefiting them in a comparative sense. However, several objections found in the bioethical literature can be raised against this assumption.

If we do not accept the non-identity-affecting assumption behind the Greater Moral Obligation View, there would be no way to support such a view. In this chapter, I present, systematize, and criticize four major objections, namely, the identity objection (Section 5.1), the critique of the necessity of rGE for the child's existence (Section 5.2), the "artificially constrained future" objection (Section 5.3), and the critique of the inevitability of Preimplantation Genetic Diagnosis (PGD) (Section 5.4). I will argue that the non-identity-affecting assumption on which the Greater Moral Obligation View rests can withstand the objections considered here, implying that the moral duties proposed are legitimate or at least worthy of further discussion.

DOI: 10.4324/9781032654683-6

5.1 The Identity Objection

The Greater Moral Obligation View and its non-identity-affecting assumption assume that the numerical identity of the embryo is not affected by genetic modification. However, this is far from obvious (de Melo-Martín, 2022).

In general terms, the identity objection argues that, due to modification through rGE, the modified embryo will develop into a numerically different person from the person who would have developed had the modification not occurred. There is a vast amount of literature on whether or not rGE affects identity (DeGrazia, 2005; Elliot, 1993; Persson, 1995; Zohar, 1991). Several versions of this objection can be identified: depending on the metaphysical notion of identity that is assumed, there will be different formulations of it, which will have different implications for the prescriptions implied by the Greater Moral Obligation View. In this section, I systematize and analyze four versions that consider numerical identity as, respectively, (a) the persistence of genetic material, (b) an integrated whole, (c) a psychological continuity, and (d) an organism. Here, I am considering only those versions of the identity objection that presuppose the Origin View as a necessary condition for numerical identity. Some authors have challenged this assumption, arguing that it is not necessary for identity, and this would have implications for the Greater Moral Obligation View (Lewens, 2015; Malek, 2022; Wrigley, 2022; Żuradzki & Dranseika, 2022). In other words, according to those authors, the same numerical identity could originate from a union between different gametes. These attempts are not considered here as they deserve a separate discussion.

Before analyzing the aforementioned versions of the identity objection, it should be noted that those who only intend to defend the permissibility of rGE usually avoid dealing with the identity objection, arguing that even if the rGE changes the identity of the future individual, it would not follow that the practice should be considered morally problematic (Holtug, 2009; Holtug & Sandøe, 1996). From this perspective, rGE could be morally controversial only if the early embryo were already considered a person: a genetic modification affecting the identity would end an individual with full moral status.

Nonetheless, reflection on the embryo's identity assumes crucial importance when we investigate what prospective parents owe their progeny from a person-affecting perspective. In other words, if we want to assess the soundness of the Greater Moral Obligation View, it is essential to discuss the identity objection, bearing in mind that reasoning about the identity of an individual or an early embryo does not necessarily mean discussing its moral status, even though there are moral perspectives that assume that individuality is a sufficient condition for the existence of a person with full moral status (Ford, 2010). The Greater Moral Obligation View is not committed to supporting the view according to which the embryo is a person or has some relevant moral status; hence, the Greater Moral Obligation View is compatible with the widespread moral belief that embryos do not have moral status, and abortion is morally legitimate. Therefore, although this view considers the genetic modification of an embryo as non-identity-affecting, it should be recalled that the entity harmed or benefited is not the embryo *per se*, but the future person developed from the modified embryo.

5.1.1 Identity as the Persistence of the Genetic Material

The first version of the identity objection assumes a strict view of identity, according to which an organism could not survive *any* replacement of its parts while maintaining the same identity. Here, the persistence of the whole genome should be considered a necessary condition for preserving the identity of the embryo. Thus, because after rGE the embryo no longer possesses the same genetic material as the embryo before the modification, such a procedure cannot be considered a treatment that benefits or harms the future individual: the embryo would no longer have the same numerical identity as the future individual and, therefore, no actual person would benefit from it, but a new identity would have originated through the modification. By modifying the genome, rGE would interrupt the continuity of development between the embryo and the individual who will be born; they, not sharing the same genes, should be considered as two different entities. Therefore, the Greater Moral Obligation View should be completely rejected.

This account seems too rigid and decidedly implausible since, as Robert Elliot observes, not all the material parts of an organism are necessary for its persistence as the same individual (Elliot, 1993). To clarify this thesis, Elliot gives the following example: just as a table to which a slight modification is made does not stop being that particular table; in the same way, the early embryo does not cease to exist when a small part of its genome is modified. Considering the specific case of rGE, the practice could be effective in the near future mainly in replacing a few genes. Indeed, it is expected to provide clinical treatment, especially for monogenic diseases. In this regard, it is clear that the embryo in which the defective gene is replaced will be modified in a minimal way; just think that the human genetic heritage is made up of a number in the order of tens of thousands of genes. Therefore, a substitution of one or two genes would be marginal. Furthermore, we should observe that our DNA can slightly change over time, but it would seem controversial to claim that these changes lead to a different numerical identity.

One might reject the overly strong claim that the persistence of *all* genetic material is required and argue that only a massive modification can change the embryo's numerical identity. For instance, Cesar Palacios-González contends that the replacement of an entire sex chromosome in embryo A could end the existence of A, which would give way to embryo B of the opposite sex: this would be a non-controversial example of changing numerical identity (Palacios-González, 2021). From this interpretation of numerical identity – that is, that the numerical identity of an entity depends on how much genetic material is preserved before or after the modification – it would be possible to argue that there are rGE non-identity-affecting treatments, namely, minimal changes in the genome such as future genetic treatments for monogenetic diseases, and there may be others, at least theoretically, that are identity affecting. We have a sorites puzzle here and, accordingly, some undecidable cases in which we will not be able to assess if the identity of the embryos has changed are inevitable.

However, this does not mean we cannot determine the identity of the embryos before and after the modification. Adding or subtracting a small proportion of matter is consistent with material continuity, although it is impossible to specify this proportion precisely. In any case, according to the revised account of the persistence of the genetic material, the Greater Moral Obligation View cannot be definitively rejected. Nevertheless, it would apply only to cases involving minor genetic changes and not to those involving more extensive ones, since the existence or absence of moral constraints toward the progeny would depend on the extent of the genetic modification.

5.1.2 Identity as an Integrated Whole

Another version of the identity objection is based on an account of identity that does not focus so much on the extent of the change of genetic material, but rather on the *effects* of the latter on the functioning of the individual. Noam Zohar argues that it is not the replacement of the genetic material that determines the alteration of identity, but a modification that causes an alteration of both the brain development and the physical characteristics of the future individual (Zohar, 1991). Identity here is not understood as the sum of the components of an entity but as an integrated whole. What differentiates the sum of the parts, such as the individual genes, and the idea of an integrated whole is that genetic makeup is conceived as the blueprint of a person's organization and functional capabilities: the way in which the parts are integrated.

By adopting a functionalist perspective on identity, Zohar believes that genetic organization is the essence of personal identity at the embryonic stage. Although he acknowledges that genetic heritage alone does not determine the identity of human beings – since other relevant elements, such as habits, ideas, and relationships, are also crucially important – these elements affect identity in a postnatal context and certainly not in the embryonic stage. With regard to embryos, all that determines identity is the genotype, which must be preserved in its functioning. In other words, a person's genotype is not the only important element of their identity; however, at the embryonic stage, "all we have to go by is the genotype" (Zohar, 1991, p. 283). Hence, if the way in which the genotype is expressed phenotypically is changed, then these changes would be sufficient for the destruction of the numerical identity and the creation of a new one.

So, while minor changes such as an alteration of the genome that introduces a change imperceptible to human eyes would not affect identity, avoiding a genetic disease surely does because it would affect the functioning and, therefore, the organization of the individual. Accordingly, this account is also committed to considering not only direct genetic change as relevant for the continuity of numerical identity but also epigenetic changes, which do not involve alterations in the DNA sequence, which produce some perceptible effects on the future individual.[1] This conclusion would imply an almost total inapplicability of the Greater Moral Obligation View, since the more disabling a disease, the more likely it will modify the functioning of the future individual.

Zohar's proposal, hoverer, is scarcely plausible if we observe that the phenotypic effect of some genetic information depends on environmental factors, which could also be manipulated through human action. In other words, the activation of a specific phenotypic effect for a gene often depends on epigenetic contingencies. It may seem controversial to argue that what is done by other people or, more generally, by society can determine which components of the genotype makeup one's essence (Elliot, 1993). More importantly, Zohar's thesis further implies that identity alterations depend on our *perceptual abilities* to detect phenotypic traits, which, again, is implausible (Elliot, 1993). Finally, the perspective of identity proposed by Zohar is questionable since he would not consider the distinction between the identity of an object and the identity of an organism (DeGrazia, 2005). Zohar provides an explanation of the identity of the embryo starting from the similarity with the dilemma of the Ship of Theseus, where one wonders whether a ship in which all the pieces are gradually replaced remains the same ship. According to Zohar, as already stated, the fact that it remains the same ship is due to its functional organization. However, even assuming that this holds for a ship or an inanimate object, according to David DeGrazia, it cannot be so for living beings in which the persistence of identity essentially has to do with the continuation of the same life as individuals (DeGrazia, 2005). I will discuss such a proposal when introducing the "identity as an organism" approach.

5.1.3 Identity as Psychological Continuity

The third version of the identity objection is based on the concept of identity as psychological continuity. Advocates of a psychological approach to numerical identity – namely, those who argue that an individual remains themself in light of the persistence of exclusively psychological elements of continuity (Parfit, 1984) – may claim that an rGE treatment would be an alteration of identity only if it provoked a different chain of connection and psychological continuity compared to the one that would have been created without the modification (Alonso & Savulescu, 2021).

In other words, if genetic modification caused an alteration of brain development leading to a different psychological trajectory, it would change the numerical identity. An rGE treatment that replaces a gene by blocking the development of cardiac dysfunction in the future individual would not affect identity; on the contrary, treatment aimed at avoiding congenital mental impairment would determine which numerical identity will come into the world. However, this is not always the case. A treatment that prevents the occurrence of neurodegenerative disease in adulthood – for example, some forms of Huntington's disease – would not affect numerical identity. Following this interpretation, the Greater Moral Obligation View should be confined to those genetic diseases that do not affect the psychological development of the future individual.

The psychological approach to identity is in line with our intuitions not only in many real-life circumstances but also in thought experiments where consciousness separates from the body, and for which we tend to argue that identity persists where our consciousness is present. However, this approach faces problems in accounting for identity issues precisely about the beginning of life (DeGrazia, 2005; Olson, 1997). According to several authors, the psychological approach contradicts embryology, namely, that human organisms develop as fetuses are born and continue to develop during the various stages of life. Since embryos and fetuses lack the ability to develop psychological connections, they cannot be considered numerically identical to the future individual, and this would give rise to the so-called fetus problem (Olson, 1997): if identity is a matter of continuity of mental contents, and no person is psychologically continuous with the embryo or fetus from which they develop, then an individual has never been the fetus from which they develop. From this, it would become difficult to justify the existence of harm or benefit not only in the context of the rGE – even if this, we assume, does not cause a different psychological structure to the future individual – but also in the context of possible harm to a fetus, when the mother deliberately takes drugs or alcohol during pregnancy. In both cases, no actual person is being harmed, neither future nor current.

To avoid these counterintuitive outcomes inherent in the psychological approach, Nicola Jane Williams recognizes that the fetus or embryo cannot be considered to be numerically identical to the future individual; however, she also observes that the embryo or fetus possesses distinctive characteristics, which are necessary for the existence of a particular future individual (Williams, 2013). From a psychological perspective, these properties determine some distinctive psychological traits in the future individual A, who could not exist as A without them. Therefore, we can continue to speak of identity, albeit in a different but still compatible way with the sense of identity we use to discuss harms and benefits. In other words, the existence of harm and benefit should no longer be sought by asking the question: "does the embryo have the same numerical identity as the future individual after the genetic modification?"; instead, one should ask: "does the embryo after the genetic modification still possess the distinctive causal characteristics that were necessary for the existence of the individual who would have been born if this modification had not occurred?". Consequently, if these distinctive characteristics remained fixed during the genetic modification process, a proponent of the psychological approach may consider an rGE treatment as a non-identity affecting practice – therefore subject to the Greater Moral Obligation View – and not one that changes the person's numerical identity. However, even with such a specification, the psychological approach would not be able to justify a moral obligation against rGE intervention that causes cognitive deficit to the future individual, or the duty not to use drugs or alcohol during pregnancy which leads to mental cognitive impairment in the newborn[2], assuming that the resulting psychological changes are sufficiently large to change identity.

Furthermore, one may reasonably ask whether it is really possible to isolate the distinctive psychological traits of an individual. While this is intuitive when comparing a person with cognitive impairment and a person without it, in other situations, it is problematic. Ingmar Persson proposes the following example: suppose a mother, immediately after giving birth, had her child adopted by a family from a different social class or in another country. Or, even worse, imagine she let him fall, causing damage to the brain such severe that the child will suffer from severe mental impairment for the rest of his life. There is probably no psychological trait that unites these three scenarios; therefore, a proponent of the psychological approach would have to conclude, rather problematically, that all scenarios have generated different existing persons and consequently that the child, in the case of the fall, has not been harmed at all. However, Persson argues that people strongly tend to believe that the child in question is the same, although they live extremely different lives in the three alternative scenarios (Persson, 1995). It should also be noted, following the psychological account, that the distinctive psychological traits would not be preserved even by some medical treatments on newborns, which could cause a different psychological trajectory in the development of the individual and, therefore, cause a newborn to cease to exist; this, again, seems very questionable and rather counterintuitive since the possibility of having person-affecting reasons for treating some pathologies in very young children would be excluded.

What is important to stress here is also that the persistence of exclusively psychological elements of continuity could be affected not only by direct changes – such as avoiding or causing a cognitive deficit through rGE – but also by indirect ones. Even treatments of embryos, fetuses, and newborns that do not directly influence their cognitive sphere still influence their way of understanding the surrounding world and, therefore, their psychological trajectory. Consider Henry, a newborn affected by Infantile Onset Ascending Hereditary Spastic Paralysis (IAHSP), the main feature of which is the progressive spasticity of the muscles of the lower limbs due to dysfunction of the pyramidal tracts. Let us assume that a treatment is available to resolve this condition. While it would not directly change Henry's psychological traits, treating this disease could have a tremendous indirect impact on him. Without this disease, Henry could have had different experiences than if Henry had not been treated: in the future, he could play and have relationships with other children, have a different relationship with his parents, etc. It is reasonable to state that IAHSP can affect the character and psychological traits that Henry will develop, even if the disease and, therefore, the treatment do not have a direct impact at the brain level. But it seems rather implausible to argue that Henry is no longer Henry if he is treated. This argument has even more relevant consequences if it is also extended to possible treatments for milder diseases (e.g., neonatal diabetes) or even for operations aimed at simply correcting aesthetic defects at birth because these conditions, however slight, can have a huge impact on the child's psychological sphere.

Therefore, proponents of the psychological approach should be prepared to argue that the Greater Moral Obligation View will not apply to virtually any situation. However, such a conclusion seems at odds with the positions that some proponents of this approach are willing to defend, and it comes at the high cost of facing the numerous criticisms and implausible implications presented here.

5.1.4 Identity as an Organism

The last version of the objection is offered by the biological approach to identity. The latter argues that human beings are not essentially "embodied minds", as the psychological approach suggests, but rather "human organisms". A living human organism is an entity that belongs to the species of *Homo sapiens* and that has the ability to carry out certain vital processes. This category includes not only adults with normal functioning but also present fetuses, people with severe dementia, and patients in a vegetative state. Being human organisms does not mean it counts morally for the entire arc of their existence, but it means that an adult human animal, who is in a position to have full moral status, was undoubtedly a fetus with no or a lower moral status.

From this perspective, once a human organism begins to exist, its identity is stable enough to resist genetic or epigenetic changes, even large-scale modifications. What matters to numerical identity is that *that* individual organism continues to stay alive (DeGrazia, 2005, 2012). According to DeGrazia, most of the arguments claiming that prenatal identity is fragile confuse numerical and narrative identity and assume, rather problematically, that individuals are essentially minds or persons, without considering that throughout our lives we are subject to radical changes without ceasing to be the same organism. From this perspective, a child who has been seriously injured in a car accident that has caused mild mental impairment is not replaced by a new person. Similarly, once a human organism has a prenatal origin, it can change significantly due to genetic modifications or factors in the uterine environment, without disappearing (DeGrazia, 2012).

To assess whether or not an organism remains the same before and after rGE, we need to determine what causes a specific organism to be that particular human organism and, therefore, understand when an organism begins to exist. Identifying this ontological-conceptual moment makes it possible to define which genetic treatments affect identity and which do not. Although a plausible candidate may be conception – since the union of a specific sperm and a specific oocyte is a necessary condition for the existence of each of us – Eric Olson and DeGrazia do not consider it as the moment in which a human organism would begin to exist. Up to about two weeks after fertilization, the embryo can still divide, giving rise to two or more twins with identical DNA. During this period, the embryo would function less as a single integrated energy-using unit of the kind we call an organism and more as a set of single-celled organisms united in a contingent fashion. This is why twinning and merging remain possible.

These considerations lead some proponents of the biological approach to argue that human organisms have never been early embryos. Accordingly, interventions at this stage could affect the organism's identity, which will come into the world in a far-reaching way that changes after this stage. After gastrulation, the identity of an organism certainly becomes more robust, so much so that even an extensive genetic modification could be compatible with the preservation of numerical identity. However, before gastrulation, things are more complex, and this could have significant implications for the Greater Moral Obligation View. In fact, rGE should be performed in a phase preceding the first cell division or immediately after, to avoid mosaicism problems, or before the transfer to the uterus and gastrulation. This means that rGE would occur at a time when there is no numerical identity of the future individual yet. Accordingly, genetic changes at this stage could have disruptive consequences on the numerical identity of the future individual.

Supporters of this understanding of the biologist approach are rather vague on the extent of disruptiveness of these consequences, and they do not specify whether the same organism can originate even after an intervention on gametes or an early embryo. It is plausible to speculate that biologists may accept the thesis that the numerical identity of the early embryos depends on how much genetic material is preserved before or after the modification, regardless of the effects, or the thesis proposed by Zohar, which focuses on the phenotypic consequences that this modification can have on the physical or cognitive development of the individual.

It is possible to reply to the thesis according to which the ontological-conceptual moment of origin of the individual would occur only after gastrulation. First, the twin division of an embryo is a quite rare phenomenon, albeit more frequent in assisted reproduction (Hviid et al., 2018). In light of this, it could be argued that embryos that do not divide are numerically identical to the individuals that will develop from them. In this context, while non-twins come into existence at conception, twins come into existence at the time of twinning. DeGrazia replies that this position is committed to arguing that each twinning is a tragedy because it would mean that the original zygote no longer exists. Furthermore, we should support policies aimed at avoiding twinning (DeGrazia, 2006). However, these arguments are ineffective in the perspective adopted in this book, which assumes that the early embryo does not have a full moral status: such a reply may be effective only if the zygote were considered an entity with moral status.

Second, and more specifically, according to Matthew Liao, arguing that an entity can divide does not mean that this entity is not an individual human organism. A living amoeba has the potential to "twin" and give rise to two or more amoebas at any time. It does not follow that there was no amoeba before the division into two or more amoebas. Or, in the case of most plants, parts of a plant can be used to create another completely new one. Again, it does not follow that a distinct plant did not exist before such a procedure (Liao, 2010).

Furthermore, the fact that the embryo is still undifferentiated does not affect the possibility of already considering it a human organism. In this regard, note that the cells of most plant forms are totipotent throughout life. Does this mean that there is never a distinct plant? It would seem not. If this is true, the fact that early embryonic cells are totipotent does not affect the possibility that a particular individual may already be present, even while twinning is still possible. Finally, it is not true that the early embryo is not a coordinated organism. Scientific evidence demonstrates an exchange of information and coordination within the unicellular zygote, the multicellular zygote, and subsequently within the morula and blastocyst (Chen et al., 2018).

Such observations would at least make it plausible for biologists not to reject the position according to which the numerical identity of an individual can originate at the moment of fertilization, at least for those embryos that never split. From this, we may support the Greater Moral Obligation View applying to the vast majority of early embryos. However, this leaves questions on how the genetically modifying gametes can affect the embryo identity formed from their union. In some circumstances, if the intervention does not change the identity of the organism, the decision to treat or not those gametes with genome editing could be morally relevant, even if the individuality does not yet exist.

5.2   The Critique of the Necessity of Genome Editing for the Existence of the Modified Individual

A different objection consists in observing that rGE could neither harm nor benefit the child because the parents-to-be's *choice* to undergo rGE determines the identity of the future individual (Alonso & Savulescu, 2021; Rehmann-Sutter, 2018; Rulli, 2019; Sparrow, 2022): the latter would never have existed without the decision to employ the IVF process and rGE. If rGE cannot harm or benefit the future individual, then the Greater Moral Obligation View cannot apply.

This critique is independent of whether or not the occurrence of rGE directly modifies the numerical identity of the embryo. Regardless of this, the embryo would have been created precisely to be modified with rGE. Here, the focus is not on the modified individual who is born, but instead on the *process* that led to the birth of an individual with the modified genome: the chain of events that led to undertaking the IVF plus rGE process has, in fact, a decisive influence on defining which identity will come into the world.

To analyze this critique, let us consider the following scenario which may be one of the first clinical applications of rGE in the short term, and it will be useful also for the discussion of the other following critiques:

> Toby is homozygous for the genetic mutation causing Huntington's disease. Suppose Toby and Maria decided to have a child not affected by Huntington's disease: this is the only condition to have a child for them. Thanks to a new rGE treatment, reproducers can conceive a child biologically related to both of them without the future child having the disease. Hence, they undergo IVF, creating one or more embryos all affected by the mutation that is intended to be avoided. Consequently, Toby and Maria employ rGE to treat the genetic disease in one of the created embryos and then transfer the modified embryo into the mother's uterus. After nine months, Rachel is born free from Huntington's mutation.

The embryo from which Rachel develops was created just to be treated with rGE to avoid the Huntington's mutation, as Toby and Maria would not have undergone IVF if there had not been the possibility – thanks to rGE – to have a child biologically related to both of them without such a mutation. The availability of rGE is a necessary condition for Rachel's existence. Therefore, without the possibility of such a treatment, Rachel would never have existed because the specific union between that sexual cell from which Rachel developed would never have occurred; Toby and Maria would have decided not to procreate at all or to have a child through other reproductive techniques such as gamete donation. The couple's decision to use rGE would not have benefited Rachel since her identity directly depends on the same process (IVF plus rGE) that is supposed to benefit her. According to such a critique, if the embryo is created just to be later modified, rGE cannot be considered a non-identity-affecting practice; hence, there would be no room for the Greater Moral Obligation View.

First, we should notice that the critique leaves open the possibility that rGE may still be considered a non-identity-affecting practice. If a sterile couple underwent IVF and then through PGD discovered that the embryo produced is suffering from a severe genetic mutation hypothetically treatable with rGE,[3] then the modified embryo would still benefit as it would not have been created for the sole purpose of being modified, as it would have been created anyway; therefore, the numerical identity is independent of the will to use the rGE which is not necessary for the embryo's existence. In those cases, the Greater Moral Obligation View may still apply.

Second, I believe it is possible to respond effectively to this criticism and thus save the Greater Moral Obligation View, even in cases in which the future individual is created only to be treated with rGE. Here, I provide a detailed explanation, arguing that the proponents of such a criticism do not consider that there is a difference between the pre- and post-conception scenarios, which is morally relevant for our discussion based on the consequences-based person-affecting perspective.

In the pre-conception scenario – the scenario that occurs before the creation of *in vitro* embryos – any prospective parents' decisions do not deal with any already determined numerical identity. In fact, prospective parents' decisions in the pre-conception scenario directly affect the numerical identity of the future child. Depending on the procreative choice at this stage, the time of conception and the reproductive methods used could change, leading to a union of different gametes and, consequently, a different numerical identity. Therefore, from a consequences-based person-affecting perspective, it is not possible to observe any moral obligation toward the future individual. In other words, a child with disease D, once born through natural intercourse, cannot complain to their parents because they have decided (before conception) not to use IVF and rGE to have a child without the disease. After all, such choices would have brought a numerically different child into existence.[4]

On the contrary, in the post-conception scenario, namely, when the *in vitro* embryo already exists, the numerical identity of the future child is already determined; this fact inaugurates a change in the moral scenario. Deciding *at this new stage* to treat the embryo with rGE or not does not create a completely new numerical identity – as happened in the pre-conception scenario – but affects the future child only qualitatively.[5] Therefore, the moral reasons to be considered in the procreators' choice do change. As the context has changed, new procreative moral duties toward the future individual emerge, regardless of whether or not the designated embryo was created to be treated with rGE.

By failing to appreciate the distinction between pre- and post-conception scenarios, the supporters of the critique discussed here are not able to recognize a relevant difference between the choice of (a) creating an embryo in order to modify it with rGE and that of (b) modifying an already existing embryo before transferring it into the mother's womb. Although such decisions may have the same purpose (e.g., having a child free from a genetic disease), they happen in different contexts with different background conditions: they are not the same choice, but two different ones with different moral requirements. As I argued in Chapter 2, our moral obligations depend on what we can control: in the pre-conception scenario, we cannot provide a comparatively better existence for our future child, since any decision will determine which future child will be born; instead, in the post-conception scenario, the background conditions are different since we deal with the same numerical identity of the future child: because of rGE, now parents have unprecedented control over the quality of the future child which leads to new obligations. At this point in the process, the fact that, without the availability of the rGE, the child would not have existed seems irrelevant because choice (a) is morally independent of choice (b), since it is subject to different contextual constraints. Now the designated embryo exists, and it may have a number of possibilities for coming into existence with different lives, namely, different possible versions of its genetic inheritance. Therefore, if the procreators decide to have a child and, after IVF, recognize a specific embryo as their future child, then they not only have preferences but also have new moral obligations.

Regarding the case of Toby and Maria – who do not want to have a child with Huntington's disease – when they decide to use IVF and then rGE to have a child free of the disease, they only express a preference because they are in the pre-conception scenario where no binding consequences-based person-affecting moral obligation can apply.[6] However, after the IVF process, we can observe the existence of the embryo that will become Rachel. Thus, before the embryo transfer, Rachel is in a condition where she can benefit from rGE. Since the prospective parents are in a scenario in which they can benefit or harm Rachel, they not only have a preference for transferring that embryo only after treating it with rGE but also have significant moral reasons for doing so. The soundness of this argument is even more evident in the hypothetical case, already encountered in Chapter 4 (Section 4.4), of sadistic prospective parents who decide to have a child with some severe genetic disease. From a consequences-based person-affecting perspective, in the pre-conception scenario, the decision to employ IVF plus rGE in order to create embryos with a genetic disease is immune from moral praise or blame; however, after the existence of the embryo designated to be implanted, sadistic prospective parents face a moral obligation not to employ rGE in order to provoke a harmful genetic condition.

From this, it can be argued that even in cases where the embryo is created only to be treated with rGE, this practice can still harm or benefit the future individual; consequently, parents have a moral duty either to resort to it or to abstain from employing it.

5.3   The "Artificially Constrained Future" Objection

A critique in some ways similar to the one just presented has been proposed by Thomas Douglas and Katrien Devolder. They claim that to assess whether rGE is a non-identity-affecting practice, we need to ask what would have been the fate of that child if the parents had decided not to undertake rGE (Douglas & Devolder, 2022). According to the authors, the morally relevant counterfactuals to assessing whether genome editing harms or benefits the future individual concern the parents' will in the case in which it is not possible to undertake rGE. In other words, the future individual cannot be benefited or harmed by rGE if parents guarantee the individual the only possible alternative future to non-existence. In this case, the future individual could not exist in any counterfactual scenario, since the parents would not have brought her into existence except in the condition in which she find herself.

We can appreciate both similarities and differences with the critique of the necessity of rGE. On the one hand, in Toby and Maria's case, the two critiques likely agree that Rachel was not benefited, since the couple, if it had not been possible to use the rGE, would not even have created the embryo and, therefore, there would have been no individual. On the other hand, things are different when we consider again the hypothetical case in which the sterile couple discovers only after the embryo exists that it is affected by a mutation that could lead to a genetic disease: according to the critique of the necessity of rGE discussed above, genetic modification is non-identity-affecting because the embryo was not initially created to be modified. According to Douglas and Devolder, instead, whether rGE is non-identity-affecting depends on the following question: in what condition would this individual have been otherwise? If the parents, in the scenario that rGE was unavailable, did not want to continue the pregnancy process by transferring that specific embryo into the uterus, then rGE would be an identity-affecting practice; on the contrary, if the parents-to-be had wanted to continue *in any case* with the transfer of that particular embryo despite its condition, rGE would still be a non-identity-affecting practice, since the individual would have existed regardless of the modification. In the former case, the only counterfactual scenario to be considered is non-existence and not the other possible alternatives in which the future individual may exist with different genes thanks to rGE. Therefore, prospective parents artificially construct the only alternative scenario in which that embryo can develop into an actual person.

According to Douglas and Devolder, in this context, the genetically modified child, similar to a genetically selected child with PGD, could not express any complaints toward the parents. Harm and benefit are comparative concepts; thus, the possibility of expressing complaints about one's genetic condition depends on the fact that the individual could have been different from how she is, namely, she could have lived a life with different genetic characteristics from those she possesses in the condition in which she finds herself. However, the authors argue that the modified individual could not have been different from what she actually is, since the only alternative to existence with this genome, according to the parents' decision, would be non-existence.

Embracing the implication of the "artificially constrained future" objection leads to a surprising conclusion: the more severe the disorder that prospective parents wish to avoid in their child, the less likely the eradication of the disease will benefit the future individual. This is because the parents are more likely not to have wanted the child with a severe genetic disorder. Conversely, rGE is more likely to benefit the future individual when used for less severe disorders (Douglas & Devolder, 2022).

The objection provided by Douglas and Devolder is controversial since it does not seem to offer any reason to consider morally relevant only the alternative worlds coinciding with the will of the parents, while excluding other possible alternatives. Moreover, accepting Douglas and Devolder's argument may have extremely counterintuitive outcomes. For example, it might support the belief that modifying an embryo to make the future individual develop a severe genetic disease, even if compatible with a life worth living, is not at all harmful to the child if this condition is the only one that parents consider possible for her existence. Hence, Douglas and Devolder are committed to arguing that, in this case, the individual would not have existed, except as suffering from a serious genetic disease.

The authors seem to confuse two distinct propositions with different moral implications: (1) the child could not have existed in a condition other than the one in which she finds herself, and (2) the parents did not want the child to exist in a different condition than the one in which she is. As for (1), the individual is in the only possible condition because there is no alternative world in which she can exist with a different condition. For example, a person affected by Trisomy 21 cannot exist without this syndrome, since it is in no way possible to treat this condition: being affected by Trisomy 21 is, therefore, a necessary condition for her existence. As for (2), the child is in a condition that would have been *technically* avoidable, namely, under the prospective parents' control: in Toby and Maria's case, Rachel could have existed with Huntington's disease, but the parents decided to avoid this condition using rGE; similarly, in the case of sadistic prospective parents, the resulting child could have existed free from the genetic severe disease, but the parents wanted simply otherwise. The severe genetic disease is not a necessary condition for the existence of that child, if not from the questionable voluntarist parent's perspective supported by the authors.

Douglas and Devolder's argument produces a moral short circuit, according to which counterfactual scenarios should be compared to assess if the future child has been harmed or not and, consequently, the morality of the parents' actions or omissions, but such scenarios are voluntarily decided by the same people who carry out the actions or omissions under moral scrutiny. The action is considered harmful, beneficial, or neutral in light of the alternatives desired by the parents. In this way, a killer who wants to kill an old lady, but then changes their mind at the last moment and shoots her in the leg can claim that they have done nothing morally deplorable as there were only two morally relevant alternatives for the old lady:[7] (a) being killed and (b) getting a bullet in the leg. One could even go further, arguing that not only did the killer not carry out a morally wrong action, but actually benefited the elderly lady. Since in (b) the elderly lady is in a better situation than in (a), she would, in fact, benefit from the killer's action, as the only counterfactual conditions were (a) and (b).

It is hard to embrace the conclusion that the killer benefited the old lady, especially if you contrast this scenario with the case of an unlucky driver who, through no fault of their own, has only enough time to run over the old lady killing her or swerve lightly and breaking her legs. In this case, since there are actually only two possibilities, we would be happy enough to say they did the right thing.

In the old lady's case, instead, there are many options open to the killer who, however, has artificially limited the morally relevant counterfactuals to only two.[8] In other words, Douglas and Devolder provide no explanation as to why the killer cannot consider the alternative in which (c) the old lady is neither killed nor injured. I believe that alternative (c) is morally relevant and provides reasons for the killer to avoid (a) and (b): the old lady could have existed in scenario (c) where she would have been better off compared to (a) and (b); the possibility of (c) existed independently of the killer's decision to unduly restrict the possible alternatives to (a) and (b); in light of this, the decision of which counterfactuals to consider in order to assess whether or not the killer harms the old lady cannot depend on the will of the killer, but instead must rely on the ability of the killer to control the occurrence of (a), (b) and (c).

Similarly, when Toby and Maria decide to have a child through IVF, and rGE is available, as they are about to transfer *in utero* the embryo that will develop in Rachel, they face at least two options: (d) Rachel without Huntington's disease and (e) Rachel with Huntington's disease. In both scenarios, Rachel can exist since (d) and (e) are *technically* possible given the material and technological capacities of the prospective parents to choose one of them. The prospective parents' decision to artificially restrict the counterfactual scenarios to only (d) does not dismiss the moral relevance of both scenarios – (d) and (e) – in order to evaluate, through a comparison, in which scenario the future person is harmed or not.

It would not even make sense to speak of morality if the actions of an agent were judged harmful, beneficial, or neutral – and therefore legitimate or not – based on the only alternatives that the agent wants to consider and not those they can consider. What makes counterfactuals morally relevant for evaluating the occurrence of harm or benefit for a subject depends on both the actual conditions of existence of the subject in the different alternative scenarios and the material capabilities of the agent who, through their actions or omissions, can actualize a scenario rather than another in which the subject may be harmed or benefited. Both aspects are independent of the will of the agent. This allows us to consider from a moral point of view what actions prospective parents *could* have performed and not just those they would have liked to have done otherwise.[9]

In light of this, it seems plausible to reject this criticism, arguing that rGE could harm or benefit the future child even if she were in the only future that parents consider possible for her.[10] The fact that future parents can choose between different possible futures for their future children creates reasons for adhering to the stronger moral requirements of the Greater Moral Obligation View.

5.4 The Critique of the Inevitability of Preimplantation Genetic Diagnosis

The last critique I discuss observes that the Greater Moral Obligation View, as well as the "artificially constrained future" objection, erroneously assumes that it would be possible to create, modify the genome, and then proceed with the transfer into the uterus of a single embryo, which is highly unlikely from a technical point of view when considering the foreseeable development of rGE in the near future. In all likelihood, the first clinical applications of rGE will involve creating and modifying more embryos and then selecting those to be transferred via PGD to avoid the already-mentioned problems of mosaicism. According to Robert Sparrow, this would bring out good reasons to claim that rGE cannot yet be considered purely non-identity-affecting and, accordingly, the Greater Moral Obligation View should be rejected (Sparrow, 2022).

This is not a conceptual argument against the Greater Moral Obligation View but a technical one, since it does not focus on the argument itself but on the practical conditions for its application. To this, some might reply that the continuous development of Assisted Reproductive Technologies (ARTs) could ultimately lead to a future context in which only one *in vitro* embryo is produced, modified, and transferred; if this scenario occurred, the supporters of the critique of the inevitability of PGD would be committed to accepting the Greater Moral Obligation View. It is also true, however, that this scenario may never occur, and this would render the Greater Moral Obligation View redundant. In what follows, I offer an independent response to this critique.

I argue that the fact that more embryos are created, selected, and even transferred in the reproductive process does not negate the obligations parents have toward the future child. In order to see this, we can consider both the future child's perspective and the parents' perspective during the procreative process.

With regard to the former, the child born after the IVF process where rGE was available would, in any case, have been in a position to be benefited or harmed by this practice and therefore would have grounds for complaint against the parents, if they had used rGE improperly or had not used it at all. This specific individual could have existed with a different genome from the one they came into the world with. Regardless of whether they are the result of selection, the embryo from which it developed was in a position where it could have been modified. This seems enough for the Greater Moral Obligation View to stand. Although Sparrow admits that, from the perspective just presented, rGE may be considered non-identity-affecting (Sparrow, 2022), he unduly forces us to focus on the *process* that led to the birth of an individual with the modified genome. However, he does not provide reasons why we should accept such a shift in order to assess our moral obligation toward the future child within the IVF process, which seems perfectly plausible as defined by the Greater Moral Obligation View.

This position is also defensible if we consider the point of view of the prospective parents. Consider again the case of Toby and Maria who undergo IVF and create several embryos. According to the Greater Moral Obligation View, knowing that every embryo will have the mutation provoking Huntington's disease, they should treat at least the embryo that they are going to transfer *in utero*. Critics observe that in order to avoid transferring an embryo with mosaicism, we need to modify more embryos and then test them with PGD to choose the embryo(s) to transfer. Therefore, parents would not have any obligation toward the future child because they do not know the identity of the child which depends on which embryo gets transferred. Nevertheless, it is perfectly plausible to argue that parents have some obligation toward their future child even if they do not yet know the future child's identity among the modified embryos selected and transferred *in utero*. Whatever the identity of the future child will be, surely a specific individual will develop that could have existed in a different situation than the one in which they actually do. To understand this point, consider a terrorist who shoots randomly into the crowd, not knowing whom they will kill; from a consequences-based person-affecting perspective, such behavior still seems wrong even if there is no willingness to hit a specific target, as it is entirely plausible that the hail of bullets will hit at least one specific individual who is entitled to complain about the behavior of the terrorist.[11]

In light of this, the argument that rGE will require selective practices in the foreseeable future fails to demonstrate that genetic modification on early embryos is an identity-affecting practice. Therefore, it fails to dismiss the procreative obligation to ensure the designated embryo(s) for transfer protection from potentially harmful – and treatable via rGE – conditions.

However, Sparrow's argument may still establish that, after having modified the embryos, prospective parents do not have a moral obligation but only a preference to transfer only those embryos in which the modification has occurred effectively. Suppose, for instance, that Toby and Maria decide – after modifying all the viable embryos to secure the future child from Huntington's disease – to transfer into the uterus three embryos to maximize the likelihood of having a child: in one of them, the genetic modification occurred perfectly, and there is no sign of mosaicism; instead, in the others, there are some problems of mosaicism. Is this choice morally wrong?

We may argue that at the moment of the decision, there is no possible alternative genome for all three embryos; all that could be done by the parents to avoid harmful conditions in the future child has actually been done. Hence, if the future individual developed from those embryos has a life worth living, there is no person-affecting reason to decide to transfer only the embryo with no mosaicism, but only a preference.

More specifically, we may argue that the resulting child with mosaicism cannot complain to the parents provided they are in a condition that is still better than the one they would have been without the modification via rGE. Consider, for instance, modification for a catastrophic single-gene disorder. Several genetic disorders, such as BRAT1, JAM3, and PHGDH, are lethal in the neonatal period, so for embryos with such mutations, rGE is potentially lifesaving. According to Julian Savulescu and Peter Singer, the expected harm of mosaicism is arguably no worse than the fate of the unedited embryos if they were implanted (Savulescu & Singer, 2019).

A more complex issue is whether the child's condition after modification was worse than a condition with the initial genetic disease, though still compatible with a life worth living. It is beyond the scope of the book to discuss this complex issue; here, I just claim that if rGE is reasonably considered safe and effective (e.g., low mosaicism risk and off-target risks), parents still have a *prima facie* moral obligation to modify all embryos that could be candidates for transfer to the uterus; in this way, every possible future individual would have a chance to be free from potentially harmful genetic diseases, such as Huntington's disease.[12]

Notes

1 For a discussion of the effects of epigenic change on numerical identity, see Räsänen and Smajdor (2022).
2 For a discussion of prenatal harm and the psychological account of identity, see Rabenberg (2021).
3 Bear in mind the technical hurdle presented in Chapter 1 and recalled in Chapter 4.
4 This is the reason why, when – as stated in Chapter 4 – only consequences are considered, the Greater Moral Obligation View leads to endorse the Mild

Restriction of Procreative Autonomy, according to which only prospective parents already within the IVF process face new moral obligations.

5 Since the critique of the necessity of rGE for the existence of the modified individual is an independent critique of the identity objection, here we put in brackets the latter.

6 It is important to note again that this claim stands from a consequences-based person-affecting perspective only. In Chapter 7, I will consider the Greater Moral Obligation View also from a non-consequences-based person-affecting perspective.

7 This case is similar to the one discussed in Feinberg (1986) and represents a version of the so-called Pre-emption Problem faced by the counterfactual comparative account of harm and benefit. For a discussion, see Johansson and Risberg (2019).

8 I am indebted to Gary O'Brien for the example of the unlucky driver.

9 For a similar argument, see Roberts (2007).

10 This is not the only way to reject the artificially constrained future objection. For instance, Savulescu and Alonso argue that "it is wrong to import a counterfactual that applies to a world where gene editing does not exist to evaluate an action in a world where it does exist". See Savulescu and Alonso (2022, p. 25).

11 This example may be found in Kahane (2009).

12 Although in this chapter I have focused on rGE, these criticisms can also be relevant for other non-identity-affecting ARTs discussed in Chapter 4. For example, Mitochondrial Replacement Therapy (MRT) via pronuclear transfer is certainly exposed to the critique of the necessity of rGE for the child's existence, the "artificially constrained future" objection, and the critique of the inevitability of Preimplantation Genetic Diagnosis. However, I believe that, as with rGE, these criticisms are ineffective in arguing that MRT via pronuclear transfer affects the identity of the future individual. The identity objection may also apply because mitochondrial DNA is actually replaced in the embryo, but probably to a marginal extent compared to that discussed for genetic modification via rGE. It is interesting to consider the identity objection also regarding other techniques that do not require IVF, namely, *in vivo* genome editing and fetal therapy. While this criticism may apply, it would become less problematic for some of its versions as the changes could be less disruptive in the later stages of embryo and fetus development. Furthermore, assuming the biologist account of identity, there would no longer be a need to justify that the early embryo is the same organism as the future individual. In fact, the modification would occur in a subsequent phase to the moment in which twinning is possible, a stage where there is more consensus among authors who support this identity account to assert that such an entity is numerically identical to the future person. Regardless of these considerations, further discussion is needed about these ARTs and the criticisms I have raised in this chapter.

References

Alonso, M., & Savulescu, J. (2021). He Jiankui's gene-editing experiment and the non-identity problem. *Bioethics, 35*(6), 563–573.

Chen, Q., Shi, J., Tao, Y., & Zernicka-Goetz, M. (2018). Tracing the origin of heterogeneity and symmetry breaking in the early mammalian embryo. *Nature Communications, 9*(1). https://doi.org/10.1038/s41467-018-04155-2

de Melo-Martín, I. (2022). Human genome editing and identity: The precariousness of existence and the abundance of argumentative options. *The American Journal of Bioethics: AJOB, 22*(9), 18–20.

DeGrazia, D. (2005). *Human identity and bioethics.* Cambridge University Press.

DeGrazia, D. (2006). Moral status, human identity, and early embryos: A critique of the President's approach. *The Journal of Law, Medicine & Ethics: A Journal of the American Society of Law, Medicine & Ethics, 34*(1), 49–57, 4.

DeGrazia, D. (2012). *Creation ethics: Reproduction, genetics, and quality of life.* Oxford University Press.

Douglas, T., & Devolder, K. (2022). Gene editing, identity and benefit. *The Philosophical Quarterly, 72*(2), 305–325.

Elliot, R. (1993). Identity and the ethics of gene therapy. *Bioethics, 7*(1), 27–40.

Feinberg, J. (1986). Wrongful life and the counterfactual element in harming. *Social Philosophy and Policy, 4*(1), 145–178.

Ford, N. (2010). *When did I begin?* Cambridge University Press. https://doi.org/10.1017/cbo9780511623554

Holtug, N. (2009). Who cares about identity? In M. A. Roberts & D. T. Wasserman (Eds.), *Harming future persons* (pp. 71–92). Springer Netherlands.

Holtug, N., & Sandøe, P. (1996). Who Benefits? – Why personal identity does not matter in a moral evaluation of germ-line gene therapy. *Journal of Applied Philosophy, 13*(2), 157–166.

Hviid, K. V. R., Malchau, S. S., Pinborg, A., & Nielsen, H. S. (2018). Determinants of monozygotic twinning in ART: A systematic review and a meta-analysis. *Human Reproduction Update, 24*(4), 468–483.

Johansson, J., & Risberg, O. (2019). The preemption problem. Philosophical Studies, *176*, 351–365.

Kahane, G. (2009). Non-identity, self-defeat, and attitudes to future children. *Philosophical Studies, 145*(2), 193–214.

Lewens, T. (2015). *The biological foundations of bioethics.* Oxford University Press.

Liao, S. M. (2010). Twinning, inorganic replacement, and the organism view. *Ratio, 23*(1), 59–72.

Malek, J. (2022). Reconceptualizing identity and ethics in the context of conception. *The American Journal of Bioethics: AJOB, 22*(9), 42–44.

Olson, E. (1997). *The human animal.* Oxford University Press.

Palacios-González, C. (2021). Reproductive genome editing interventions are therapeutic, sometimes. *Bioethics, 35*(6), 557–562.

Parfit, D. (1984). *Reasons and persons.* Oxford University Press.

Persson, I. (1995). Genetic therapy, identity and the person-regarding reasons. *Bioethics, 9*(1), 16–31.

Rabenberg, M. (2021). Prenatal injury and the nonidentity problem. *Canadian Journal of Philosophy, 51*(2), 123–142.

Räsänen, J., & Smajdor, A. (2022). Epigenetics, harm, and identity. *The American Journal of Bioethics: AJOB, 22*(9), 40–42.

Rehmann-Sutter, C. (2018). Why human germline editing is more problematic than selecting between embryos: Ethically considering intergenerational relationships.

The New Bioethics: A Multidisciplinary Journal of Biotechnology and the Body, *24*(1), 9–25.

Roberts, M. A. (2007). The non-identity fallacy: Harm, probability and another look at Parfit's depletion example. *Utilitas, 19*(3), 267–311.

Rulli, T. (2019). Reproductive CRISPR does not cure disease. *Bioethics, 33*(9), 1072–1082.

Savulescu, J., & Alonso, M. (2022). Is gene editing harmless? Two arguments for gene editing. *The American Journal of Bioethics: AJOB, 22*(9), 23–28.

Savulescu, J., & Singer, P. (2019). An ethical pathway for gene editing. *Bioethics, 33*(2), 221–222.

Sparrow, R. (2022). Human germline genome editing: On the nature of our reasons to genome edit. *The American Journal of Bioethics: AJOB, 22*(9), 4–15.

Williams, N. J. (2013). Possible persons and the problem of prenatal harm. *The Journal of Ethics, 17*(4), 355–385.

Wrigley, A. (2022). Modality and counterfactuals: Understanding the role and context of metaphysical underpinnings for harm, benefit and identity claims arising from genome editing and genetic modification. *The American Journal of Bioethics: AJOB, 22*(9), 52–54.

Zohar, N. J. (1991). Prospects for "genetic therapy" – can a person benefit from being altered? *Bioethics, 5*(4), 275–288.

Żuradzki, T., & Dranseika, V. (2022). Reasons to genome edit and metaphysical essentialism about human identity. *The American Journal of Bioethics: AJOB, 22*(9), 34–36.

6 Responsibility, Genetic Enhancement, and the Child's Right to an Open Future[1]

In the previous chapter, I defended the non-identity-affecting assumption of the Greater Moral Obligation View against four important critiques. This implies that the moral obligations entailed by this view are legitimate or, at the very least, worthy of further discussion. As I have argued, accepting the Greater Moral Obligation View in the context in which reproductive Genome Editing (rGE) is available leads us to endorse the Mild Restriction of Procreative Autonomy, when considering a consequences-based person-affecting perspective. However, this is a procreative-parental responsibility model that we might define as "negative", in the sense that it requires prospective parents only to avoid genetic disease leading to disability in the future individuals. I proposed this formulation first because the Mild Restriction of Procreative Autonomy primarily aims to assess *when* moral obligations toward offspring arise, rather than exhaustively specifying the content of such duties. Second, there are important inclusivity reasons: this model does not claim to provide a complete definition of procreative-parental responsibility, but to justify prescriptions that people with different moral perspectives could accept. It is precisely for this reason that I limited the definition of what I consider harm to genetic conditions that lead to both (a) significant impairment of physical and mental well-being and (b) significant reduction of rights and opportunities accessible to an individual, allowing for the choice between a reasonable range of different life plans. From this perspective, I argued that some genetic diseases can be harmful in both (a) and (b) terms, highlighting a moral obligation to avoid these conditions in the future individual. However, some might argue that procreative responsibility, like parental responsibility, consists not only in refraining from harming the future individual or protecting them from conditions that satisfy criteria (a) and (b) but also in promoting their interests, autonomy, and well-being in ways that extend beyond conditions previously considered harmful (Glover, 2006). In this direction, Sergio Filippo Magni proposes the Principle of Person-Affecting Procreative Beneficence, which, although overlapping with the Minimal Threshold Model in a

DOI: 10.4324/9781032654683-7

context in which only selective Assisted Reproductive Technologies (ARTs) are used, has morally relevant implications in the context of rGE or the other non-identity-affecting ARTs. Indeed, Magni argues that it is morally mandatory to give the best possible life to the specific future child, maximizing their well-being (Magni, 2021). In this case, there would also be positive duties in the procreative context that would also include genetic enhancement. As a matter of fact, as argued in Chapter 1, the future availability of rGE and other non-identity-affecting techniques might not only allow the avoidance of certain genetic diseases but also improve some future individual traits. Although it is hard to provide a clear definition, here I define genetic enhancement as using ARTs in the following ways: (1) to improve capabilities or modify traits – like intelligence, height, and memory – in embryos that would already develop into a person possessing the characteristics for normal human functioning (Douglas, 2015); and (2) to modify aesthetic traits of the progeny, such as hair or eye color.

Due to this, to provide a complete picture of moral obligations that fall within the sphere of procreative-parental responsibility highlighted by the Greater Moral Obligation View, we should go beyond the discussion carried out in Chapter 4, in which I focused only on avoiding the potentially harmful genetic conditions in the future child, and also consider how prospective parents should act in light of the availability of genetic enhancement. As briefly mentioned in Chapter 4 (Section 4.5), the availability of genetic enhancement has some implications for reproductive responsibility prescriptions. However, here I focus specifically on procreative-parental responsibility.

In the discussion, I will mainly refer to rGE for argumentative convenience because this technology constitutes the main focus of the book. Nonetheless, these reflections may also be valid for other non-identity-affecting ARTs. Obviously, as far as rGE is concerned, the provisions of the Mild Restriction of the Procreative Autonomy relating to the circumstances in which the procreative duty arises remain valid: any duty of future parents to improve their child would emerge only when they are already within the *In Vitro* Fertilization process. For other techniques that affect the person, such as *in vivo* gene therapy or fetal therapy, the obligations may also extend to other contexts indicated in Chapter 4 (Subsection 4.4.3).

Addressing procreative responsibility in the context of genetic enhancement is undoubtedly complex, and it is not possible to offer an exhaustive discussion here: to do so, it would be appropriate, stemming from the criteria we used to discuss which conditions should be considered a harm for the future child, to evaluate which one is more important, namely, which is lexically priority. In other words, we should ask whether it is more important to promote well-being or open opportunities. While there may be overlap in many situations, there may be conflicts especially in the field of genetic enhancement.

This conflict may arise both when considering the future child alone – for example, modifying a trait might increase well-being but restrict rights and opportunities – and when considering the balance between the interests of the future parent and the future individual – for instance, the child's interest in having a modified trait that produces a great deal of well-being could conflict with the parents' autonomy to procreate under certain conditions. It seems we have a conflict of different values, and comparing them may be as difficult as comparing apples and oranges (Davis, 2010). To avoid these problems, in this chapter I will only consider genetic enhancement as a tool for promoting opportunities, which are ultimately a matter of autonomy. In this way, it will be easier to evaluate how to balance the interests at stake, in particular between those of the future child and those of the prospective parent. In this context, a promising tool to frame our reflection is the Child's Right to an Open Future (CROF) argument, already presented in Chapter 2 with regard to parental responsibility.[2]

According to CROF, parents should ensure the future autonomy and self-realization of their children. There is broad consensus that genetic modifications to eradicate diseases align with CROF's requirements. However, the same does not hold true for genetic enhancements. Some authors reject the claim that CROF might permit genetic enhancement (Mintz et al., 2019), others argue that CROF should only allow specific types of enhancement (Agar, 2004; Buchanan et al., 2000), and still others even believe that CROF justifies a moral obligation to genetically improve future progeny (Resnik, 2000; Savulescu, 2009; Schmidt, 2007). The disagreement over the conclusions drawn from the same argument seems to make CROF a poor tool for informing procreative choices in the field of genetic enhancement. In light of this, it becomes necessary to analyze such disagreement to propose a revised version of the argument and thus assess how procreative-parental responsibility changes in light of the availability of genetic enhancement.

The chapter is structured as follows. First, in Section 6.1, I will analyze the CROF version proposed by Dena Davis; then in Section 6.2, I will address the argument that CROF is against any type of enhancement. After rejecting this argument, maintaining that CROF is not necessarily in contrast with some genetic enhancements, in Section 6.3, I will discuss a second argument, which claims that CROF not only contrasts with some genetic improvements but also morally requires them. Therefore, I will argue that future parents do not have the moral obligation to open as many opportunities as possible for their children, but should rather aim to provide them with a reasonable range of opportunities. In light of this, in

Section 6.4, I will recognize that the moral obligations required by CROF directly depend on the dominant cooperative framework. Therefore, in Section 6.5, I will conclude that, at present, prospective parents are not morally obligated to genetically enhance their children as an unenhanced person already has access to a reasonable range of opportunities. However, the moral obligation to enhance progeny might arise if a structural change in the dominant cooperative framework were to occur.

6.1   Procreative Choices and the Child's Right to an Open Future

As already stated in Chapter 2, one of the most debated arguments to define parental responsibility is undoubtedly CROF. From this perspective, children have rights-in-trust, which cannot be exercised during childhood and, therefore, must be preserved until they become adults. In light of this, CROF requires that "children's basic options be kept open and growth be natural or unforced" (Feinberg, 1980, p. 127). In other words, it involves preserving the right to anticipatory autonomy, a right attributable to adults but that must be safeguarded during a child's childhood for future exercise. In addition, parental choices that could have definitive and irreversible consequences for the child should be avoided until they can make their own life plan decisions.

Although CROF was primarily proposed to guide parental choices regarding child-rearing, it is an argument often used in the procreative context as well. Davis claims that not only parental choices made after the birth of the baby can violate the child's right to an open future but also decisions made before birth. Specifically, procreative choices in the context of PGD, namely, selecting embryos according to the genetic traits, might confine the future child forever to a narrow group of people and a limited set of careers. Davis analyzes the aforementioned case of deaf prospective parents who want to give birth to a deaf child: prospective parents who employ PGD to select for deafness violate CROF since "they are deliberately constraining the ability of their children to make a wide variety of choices when they become adults" (Davis, 2010, p. 84).[3] According to Davis, this conclusion is consistent with both interpretations of deafness, namely, deafness as a disability (Harris, 2000) and as a cultural trait (Sparrow, 2005). Indeed, regardless of the interpretation we support, prospective parents limit cultural, social, and career choices, since such a choice forecloses significant pieces of the child's adult life and cannot normally be reversed during the child's life (Davis, 2010). In this way, the future child would not be able to lead a lifestyle grounded in values that differ substantially from those of their parents. The formulation provided by Davis suggests some moral limitations on the Principle of Procreative

Autonomy primarily in order to deliberately avoid constraining, through genetic selection, the ability of the future child to make a wide variety of choices when they become an adult. In light of the arguments presented in the previous chapters, it is evident that Davis assumes an impersonal definition of harm. However, in this context, CROF is intended to be applied only to the possibility of modifying embryos and fetuses with rGE or other non-identity-affecting techniques discussed in Chapter 4 (Subsection 4.4.3). From this perspective, the requests of Davis's proposal are compatible with those of the Mild Restriction of Procreative Autonomy presented in Chapter 4. Nonetheless, it remains unclear how CROF can inform procreative choices in light of the availability of genetic enhancement through rGE.

6.2   Closing the Door to an Open Future?

Some CROF advocates claim that all kinds of genetic enhancement should be considered inconsistent with CROF. According to Rachel Mintz and colleagues, rGE for enhancing aims undermines CROF because such a practice compromises the autonomy of the future child (Mintz et al., 2019). With rGE, anticipatory autonomy rights of the future individual would not be preserved but would rather be taken over by the parents' preferences. To establish whether or not the right to have a non-enhanced genome should be considered as a right-in-trust, the authors consider the features of personhood that develop in children as they mature (Feinberg, 1980): (1) abilities of self-governance necessary for autonomy; (2) skills or acquired abilities; (3) options or opportunities; and (4) preferences based upon desires and values. Mintz and colleagues maintain that if one considers germline engineering in light of Joel Feinberg's four features of personhood, the child's potential to exercise autonomy is preserved only if we postpone such treatments. Autonomy is more important than any capacity that can be provided through germline engineering other than life itself (Mintz et al., 2019). Furthermore, at the time when rGE is viable, namely, at the *in vitro* stage, prospective parents cannot know what capacities, options, skills, or preferences the future individual will want to have. Therefore, genetic manipulation might be unnecessary, since one could open up possibilities that the future child would not want to pursue, or at worst, it might be counterproductive, since one could risk restricting possibilities that the child would want to pursue (Mintz et al., 2019).

In short, forcing a future child into the parent's notions of the good life through genetic enhancement would likely violate CROF. From this perspective, rGE should be allowed only to save a life or mitigate a life of pain and suffering and not to enhance any trait in the future individual.

6.2.1 *Objections to the Restrictive Formulation of the Child's Right to an Open Future Argument*

This view presents some weaknesses that make it difficult to support it. First, there are numerous genetic treatments, other than those aimed at saving a life or mitigating a life of pain and suffering, which do not undermine the child's right to an open future. It is worth noting that I agree with Mintz and colleagues when they claim that providing some specific traits could undermine the development of future life's autonomy by forcing the child to follow a life plan that has been decided by their parents. For instance, modifying an embryo to obtain a child with specific personality traits is a direct infringement of CROF. Indeed, parents' wishes could convey the prejudices of a particular historical age, preventing the child from having an open future. In this regard, John Mackie states: "If the Victorians had been able to use genetic engineering, they would have made us more pious and patriotic" (Mackie cited in Glover, 1984, p. 149). However, it does not follow that *every* kind of enhancement undermines CROF. Genetic enhancements, such as expanding the future individual's lifespan, enhancing human vision, or even improving memory or general intelligence, should not be considered against the child's open future; on the contrary, these interventions may even enlarge the range of the possible life plans of the future individual or, at least, help her to make better choices about her life (Schaefer et al., 2014).

Furthermore, contra Mintz and colleagues, it seems reasonable to maintain that CROF should also consider some aesthetic enhancements as ethically legitimate interventions. Let us consider, for instance, choosing the hair and eye color of the future individual according to the parents' preferences. While one could argue that in some cultures around the world, having some particular aesthetic traits could limit the range of life plans, in Western society, it seems quite difficult to support that view.[4] In this context, changing these traits would not necessarily close the door to an open future; hence, they should be considered morally legitimate. Here, Mintz and colleagues would reply that these kinds of aesthetic enhancements (and generally every genetic enhancement) are not in line with the second formulation of the categorical imperative provided by Immanuel Kant, according to which people should be treated not as merely means but also as ends in themselves (Kant, 1797/1993). Indeed, in their paper, Mintz and colleagues theoretically ground CROF on the second formulation of the Kantian imperative from which they derive the concept of autonomy. From this perspective, choosing the hair or eye color of the future child should be considered an instrumentalization of the embryo, which is considered a mere means to create the parent's ideal child. Given that embryo and person, such as child and adult, are interrelated biological stages of growth on the same continuum of humanity, genetically enhancing the embryo would undermine the autonomy and human dignity of the future individual.

Nevertheless, even if we accept the notion of autonomy provided by Kant, it seems quite hard to support the thesis according to which the aforementioned aesthetic enhancement should be banned. Mintz and colleagues give an overly strong interpretation of Kant's principle, making it too demanding and difficult to apply. Indeed, asking parents to adhere to such a strict application of the Kantian principle, assuming its putative plausibility, might make the growing-up process impossible. If we maintain that choosing hair or eye color is a direct infringement of the Kantian principle, many daily actions concerning the relationship between parents and children will have to be considered morally wrong as well: for instance, by choosing a dress with a specific color for a newborn, parents may be treating the child as a means for the satisfaction of having a child who dresses in a certain way; but, this seems quite bizarre.

Someone might reply that, whereas choosing a person's eye color produces a permanent state, this is not so with choosing a dress; hence, the former action should be considered more problematic (from a Kantian perspective) than the latter. However, to maintain that action is a direct infringement of the Kantian principle only if it has a permanent effect seems implausible; on the one hand, one can damage another person even without causing permanent effects (e.g., kidnapping for 48 hours somebody who suffers during that time, but who will not have future psychological problems caused by this event). On the other hand, a person can cause a permanent effect on another without exploiting her (e.g., sending children to school where they will develop cognitive capabilities that will permanently change their perceptions and abilities to interact with the world). I argue that the permanent effects of an action are neither sufficient nor necessary conditions to be aligned with the Kantian principle. In the specific context of procreation, what really matters is to avoid taking away future possibilities from the range of the individual's choices.

In sum, choosing hair or eye color, precisely as choosing a specific dress for the child, does not corrupt the possibility for parents to consider the child as an end in itself and not as a mere means. It seems more reasonable to claim that autonomy is undermined only if parents decide to provide the future child with some specific traits, constraining the future possibility of individual choices. Only in this way, do prospective parents make the child unable to live autonomously. For instance, providing a specific type of intelligence to the future individual might be considered morally objectionable for the aforementioned reasons. In line with these considerations and in agreement with several scholars, we can claim that not every genetic enhancement is inconsistent with CROF (Agar, 2004;

Buchanan et al., 2000; Mameli, 2007; Savulescu, 2009) and that the aforementioned view of this argument does not offer a satisfactory interpretation of it.

Furthermore, it is also important to add that, in agreement with Mintz and colleagues, it is nevertheless reasonable to delay enhancement interventions until an individual reaches maturity to decide for themself. However, many genetic treatments would have to be performed very early in order to be effective (Savulescu, 2009).

6.3   Genetic Enhancement: Can We or Should We?

Someone could argue that, in order to respect the future individual's right to have an open future, parents should not only avoid deliberately constraining her possibilities but also enhance her capacities. Eric Schmidt proposes a helpful metaphor to explain this position: "imagine a map containing all possible significant experiences, including but not limited to educational, vocational, aesthetic and cultural experiences" (Schmidt, 2007, p. 193). By "significant experiences", Schmidt refers to experiences that can potentially change the path of a person's future. Through genetic modification, parents can modify the child's map and so modify the child's range of open futures; they can intervene with genetic modifications that, so to say, add roads to the map, allowing the child to have significant experiences that the child could not otherwise have had. Hence, such "added roads" to the child's map would expand the child's range of open futures. Schmidt suggests that this CROF understanding provides further ethical guidance, whereas Davis's requirement of substantial constraint does not. Indeed, from this perspective, prospective parents act ethically only if they make procreative choices that expand their child's range of futures. Since some genetic enhancement, far from restricting a child's future, may increase the number of possibilities or at least the quality of the child's future (Savulescu, 2009), conceiving genetic enhancement as permissible but not morally required may not be enough. As a matter of fact, we should face a moral obligation to use enhancements as instruments to enlarge the openness of the child's future.

Such an interpretation of CROF also seems in line with Feinberg's view: as Claudia Mills suggests, he would claim that parents have a duty not to isolate children intentionally from other ways of life and to make sure that their children will learn a variety of ways of life (Mills, 2003, p. 541). CROF would, in fact, require that parents comply with both negative and positive duties toward progeny. However, claiming that CROF calls for some positive parental duties, rather than only negative ones – namely, seeking to actively provide an open future, rather than just to avoid constraining it – is not enough to claim the existence of a moral obligation to enhance their progeny. To support the existence of a moral duty to genetically enhance the progeny, we should assume a maximizing conception of CROF. According to the Maximizing View, parents have a moral obligation to open as many options as possible for the future person, namely, maximizing her possibility to make the widest variety of choices in her life because it may maximize the child's chances for self-fulfillment (Feinberg, 1980). From this perspective, genetically enhancing the progeny is a way to enlarge the child's chances for self-fulfillment, and as a consequence, parents should be morally committed to employing them.

6.3.1   Toward the Moderate Conception of CROF: Critique of the Maximizing View

I argue that the Maximizing View is difficult to embrace due to its implausible implications (Millum, 2014). First, the moral obligation to open as many options as possible forces parents to make some unrealistic assumptions about the possible future desires of their child and to give up, or at least reduce dramatically, the importance of their own ideals for their children's lives (Ruddick, 1999). Second, according to Mills, CROF in its Maximizing View is even impossible to satisfy, since parents would never be able to avoid violating the child's right to an open future (Mills, 2003). Accordingly, this approach implies a too demanding and impossible to hold neutrality about values, which can produce a sort of alienation of the child from her parents. Third, from a more practical point of view, according to Francis Kamm, the Maximizing View also bizarrely requires prospective parents to use genetic modification to alter the makeup of individuals who would naturally have an excessively constricted range of options, even if those options are very good ones (Kamm, 2005). Therefore, there seem to be good reasons to reject the Maximizing View. A more plausible interpretation of the parental duties required by CROF is the Satisfying View (Buchanan et al., 2000; Lotz, 2006) or what Joseph Millum calls the Moderate Interpretation of CROF (Millum, 2014).

From this perspective, CROF only requires that the future adult be able to choose among some, perhaps particularly important, sets of options. Negatively construed, this requires allowing the child to acquire certain skills and ensuring that certain options are not closed off. Positively construed, it requires helping the child to develop key skills and providing her with the resources to choose among a reasonable range of opportunities (Millum, 2014). By a "reasonable range of opportunities", I mean varied, relevant, and culturally meaningful options, which, in a broad sense, can be considered representative of the diversity of ways of life (Lotz, 2006). Furthermore, the Satisfying View does not call for the level of neutrality required by the Maximizing View but rather for a sort of "approximate neutrality" (Lotz, 2006). Following the Satisfying View, I argue that it is too demanding to morally oblige parents to expand their child's range of futures through genetic enhancement and that this does not constitute a reasonable interpretation of CROF. It seems sensible to claim that non-enhanced children already have a reasonable array of opportunities. However, in order to justify this claim, I must recall the concept of what Allen Buchanan calls "dominant cooperative framework".

6.4 The Reasonable Range of Opportunities and the Dominant Cooperative Framework

As already argued in Chapter 2, the "dominant institutional infrastructure for productive interaction" or, more simply, "dominant cooperative framework" is the set of basic institutions and practices that enable individuals and groups in a given society to engage in ongoing mutually beneficial cooperation (Buchanan, 1996, 2011; Buchanan et al., 2000). Participating successfully in this mutually beneficial cooperation allows people to have a reasonable range of opportunities within a society, namely, to have access to a significant number of careers, life plans, and social positions, which would not be accessible outside that framework. Indeed, most of the desires that an individual can have during her life can only be realized within a cooperative social context: in this way, we can claim that having a reasonable number of opportunities for a person depends on being included, and to what extent, in the dominant cooperative framework of a society.

The ability to perform the tasks required by the institutional rules of interaction – hence, having access to a great number of opportunities – "depends not just upon what skills and talents the individuals have, but also upon the character of the demands of the forms of interaction specified by the rules" (Buchanan, 1996, p. 40). From this perspective, choosing which rules should govern the dominant cooperative scheme means choosing who will be able to have a reasonable range of opportunities within society. As a matter of fact, an individual will be able to participate successfully in the interaction if there is a good fit between her abilities and the demands of the form of interaction (Buchanan, 1996).

Deciding which rules should guide the dominant cooperative framework within a society is a complex ethical task beyond the scope of this chapter, since I am investigating the problem only through the lens of CROF. Here, we can only observe that the rules of cooperative frameworks are usually decided by the majority of people who join them. As a consequence, if the majority of people possess specific cognitive and physical skills, it is reasonable to claim that the chosen dominant cooperative framework will require cooperators to possess the aforementioned traits to have access to the majority of careers, life plans, and social positions. It is important to notice that possessing the cognitive and physical skills of the majority of people within a society is not a sufficient condition to have access to a reasonable range of opportunities; people also need other primary goods, such as education or healthcare, to realize their life plans. However, having such traits should be considered a necessary condition, although it is neither the only nor a sufficient one.

Nowadays, the majority of people within our society have the normal, namely, non-enhanced, functioning capabilities of the human species; therefore, it is likely that the dominant cooperative framework generally shall be based on those capabilities. It would seem bizarre for the cooperative scheme in our society to require people to fly, to have an enhanced view, or to have physical and cognitive capacities and endurance above the human standard, since no one in our society possesses these traits. The aforementioned skills are just not necessary to have the possibility to realize a significant number of life plans and then have a reasonable range of opportunities. Hence, having a reasonable range of opportunities depends on the conformation of the dominant cooperative framework, which in turn depends on the functioning capabilities of the majority of human beings in a given society.

Therefore, since CROF requires that parents guarantee a reasonable range of opportunities, such a moral obligation strictly depends on the dominant cooperative framework within a specific society. As claimed above, I believe that unenhanced people – individuals who possess the normal functioning capabilities of the human species – can already join the dominant social framework and, as a consequence, can have a reasonable range of opportunities. Thus, we can justify the claim that parents who decide not to genetically enhance their child are not infringing CROF. Therefore, those enhancements in line with CROF should be considered permissible; however, this argument does not necessarily call for a moral obligation to genetically enhance the progeny.

6.5   Changing the Framework, Changing the Obligations

Linking CROF with the concept of the dominant cooperative framework allows us to provide another important consideration: cooperative frameworks change over time and, since the moral obligations toward progeny required by CROF regarding genetic enhancement depend on the dominant cooperative framework, such duties change as the dominant social framework changes.

Let us consider an example outside the topic of genetic enhancement to clarify this important point. In the past, in order to have a reasonable range of opportunities within Italian society, it was not strictly necessary to have a good knowledge of the English language. As a matter of fact, many courses of study and careers did not require such knowledge. However, in recent years, due to economic, political, and social dynamics, the English language has become a requirement for many careers and life plans; moreover, primary schools have started providing English lessons and, nowadays, a growing number of Italian people speak English as a second language.

In this context, we can appreciate a change in the dominant cooperative framework; whereas in the past, English was not required to have a reasonable range of opportunities, it is nowadays. Hence, assuming that the English language is a requirement to access a reasonable range of opportunities, nowadays CROF requires parents to enable their children to attend English lessons. On the contrary, this obligation would not have arisen in the past when the English language was not required to access a reasonable range of opportunities.

In the same way, we should offer similar considerations in the field of genetic enhancement. As I have claimed above, some genetic enhancements, such as improving memory or general intelligence, are not in contrast with CROF; hence, they should be considered ethically legitimate. As a consequence of the permissibility of such genetic enhancements and their availability, a great number of people in a society might be enhanced, and this could have some challenging consequences on the assets of the dominant cooperative framework.

Assuming a scenario in which the majority of human beings, but not all, are enhanced to have much greater cognitive abilities and significantly augmented capacity for complex practical reasoning, the interaction between enhanced people becomes more sophisticated and more productive than the interaction between non-enhanced people (Buchanan, 2011). Since the functioning capabilities of the majority of human beings in a given society determine the rules shaping the dominant cooperative framework, there is a reasonable likelihood that the framework will be transformed as the number of enhanced people increases within society. For instance, the mainstream economy and the most important political processes will be structured for enhanced people and no longer for unenhanced ones. The result is that the unenhanced people will no longer have access to a reasonable range of opportunities in a given society.

Therefore, in these specific circumstances, the moral obligations required by CROF will change compared to a situation in which the dominant cooperative framework was shaped by non-enhanced human beings. Indeed, since according to the Satisfying View of CROF we have a positive duty to guarantee a reasonable range of opportunities to our progeny, in this context, we need to enhance them because the only way to have a reasonable range of opportunities in the new dominant cooperative framework is being enhanced. In other words, the moral obligations required by CROF are fluid over time, and they might change as the dominant cooperative framework changes.

To summarize, CROF is not in contrast with genetic enhancements, as long as they do not compromise the development of the child's future life or their autonomy or confine her to a life plan decided by her parents. Genetic enhancements such as expanding the future individual's lifespan, enhancing human vision, or even improving memory or general intelligence in some cases may not be considered against the child's open future. However, it is nevertheless reasonable to delay enhancement interventions until an individual reaches maturity to decide for themselves except for those that would have to be performed very early in life to have an impact.

Furthermore, CROF requires prospective parents to not open as many options as possible to their children, but rather to provide a reasonable range of opportunities. Having a reasonable range of opportunities depends on the dominant cooperative framework, which may change over time. As a consequence, the moral obligations required by CROF change as the dominant cooperative framework changes. Therefore, CROF nowadays, within the current dominant cooperative framework, parents are not obliged to genetically enhance their children since a non-enhanced person who possesses traits within the normal functioning of the species already has access to a reasonable range of opportunities. However, if the dominant cooperative framework changed, and if it required cognitive and physical capabilities that can only be reached through genetic enhancement, then parents, in order to provide a reasonable range of opportunities for their future children, would be morally obliged to enhance them.

Notes

1 This chapter revisits and expands upon the work presented in Battisti (2020), frequently employing the same wording as the original published article.
2 Prusak has argued that the CROF is not a very useful tool for addressing issues of procreative duties in the context of genetic enhancement, since respecting the child's right to an open future may not be enough to legitimize genetic enhancement (Prusak, 2013). According to the author, CROF would fail to consider some enhancements that would violate the morally problematic parent–child relationship, rendering parents' love all too conditional. Considering only a consequences-based person-affecting perspective, where intentions are not taken into account, CROF remains an appropriate tool for the discussion proposed here. I will briefly touch upon the discussion regarding the parent–child relationship and genetic enhancement in Chapter 7 (Section 7.4), but I do not take a definitive position, leaving the debate open for further reflections.
3 For a similar argument, see Camporesi (2010).
4 Here I am referring only to aesthetic traits such as the aforementioned hair and eye color. For others, such as skin color, things are more complex. The recent, growing attention to racialization and racial inequalities suggests that having

a particular skin color could limit the range of life plans even in Western societies. In this chapter, I do not want to deal with this delicate and important issue which requires an in-depth analysis that takes into account concerns about discrimination. This topic was touched upon in Chapter 4 when presenting the Principle of Procreative Justice. For a study that analyzes race and economic opportunity in the United States, see Chetty et al. (2020).

References

Agar, N. (2004). *Liberal eugenics: In defence of human enhancement.* John Wiley & Sons.

Battisti, D. (2020). Genetic enhancement and the child's right to an open future. *Phenomenology and Mind, 19,* 212.

Buchanan, A. (1996). Choosing who will be disabled: Genetic intervention and the morality of inclusion. *Social Philosophy & Policy, 13*(2), 18–46.

Buchanan, A. (2011). *Beyond humanity?: The ethics of biomedical enhancement.* Oxford University Press.

Buchanan, A., Brock, D. W., Daniels, N., & Wikler, D. (2000). *From chance to choice.* Cambridge University Press.

Buchanan, A. E., & Brock, D. W. (2000). *Studies in philosophy and health policy: Deciding for others: The ethics of surrogate decision making.* Cambridge University Press.

Camporesi, S. (2010). Choosing deafness with preimplantation genetic diagnosis: An ethical way to carry on a cultural bloodline? *Cambridge Quarterly of Healthcare Ethics: CQ: The International Journal of Healthcare Ethics Committees, 19*(1), 86–96.

Chetty, R., Hendren, N., Jones, M. R., & Porter, S. R. (2020). Race and economic opportunity in the United States: An intergenerational perspective. *The Quarterly Journal of Economics, 135*(2), 711–783.

Davis, D. S. (2010). *Genetic dilemmas* (2nd ed.). Oxford University Press.

Douglas, T. (2015). The harms of enhancement and the conclusive reasons view. *Cambridge Quarterly of Healthcare Ethics: CQ: The International Journal of Healthcare Ethics Committees, 24*(1), 23–36.

Feinberg, J. (1980). The child's right to an open future. In W. Aiken & H. Lafollette (Eds.), *Whose child?* (pp. 124–153). Rowman & Littlefield.

Glover, J. (1984). *What sort of people should there be?* Penguin.

Glover, J. (2006). *Choosing children.* Oxford University Press.

Harris, J. (2000). Is there a coherent social conception of disability? *Journal of Medical Ethics, 26*(2), 95–100.

Kamm, F. M. (2005). *Bioethical prescription: To create, end, choose, and improve lives.* Oxford University Press.

Kant, I. (1993). *Grounding for the metaphysics of morals* (J. W. Ellington, Trans.). Hackett Publishing.

Lotz, M. (2006). Feinberg, mills, and the child's right to an open future. *Journal of Social Philosophy, 37*(4), 537–551.

Magni, S. F. (2021). In defence of person-affecting procreative beneficence. *Bioethics, 35*(5), 473–479.

Mameli, M. (2007). Reproductive cloning, genetic engineering and the autonomy of the child: The moral agent and the open future. *Journal of Medical Ethics*, *33*(2), 87–93.

Mills, C. (2003). The child's right to an open future? *Journal of Social Philosophy*, *34*(4), 499–509.

Millum, J. (2014). The foundation of the child's right to an open future. *Journal of Social Philosophy*, *45*(4), 522–538.

Mintz, R. L., Loike, J. D., & Fischbach, R. L. (2019). Will CRISPR germline engineering close the door to an open future? *Science and Engineering Ethics*, *25*(5), 1409–1423.

Prusak, B. G. (2013). *Parental obligations and bioethics*. Routledge.

Resnik, D. B. (2000). The moral significance of the therapy-enhancement distinction in human genetics. *Cambridge Quarterly of Healthcare Ethics: CQ: The International Journal of Healthcare Ethics Committees*, *9*(3), 365–377.

Ruddick, W. (1999). *Parenthood: Three concepts and a principle* (L. Houlgate, Ed.; pp. 242–51). Wadsworth.

Savulescu, J. (2009). *Genetic interventions and the ethics of enhancement of human beings*. Oxford University Press.

Schaefer, G. O., Kahane, G., & Savulescu, J. (2014). Autonomy and enhancement. *Neuroethics*, *7*(2), 123–136.

Schmidt, E. B. (2007). The parental obligation to expand a child's range of open futures when making genetic trait selections for their child. *Bioethics*, *21*(4), 191–197.

Sparrow, R. (2005). Defending deaf culture: The case of cochlear implants. *Journal of Political Philosophy*, *13*(2), 1467–9760.

7 Beyond Consequences? Attitudes and Intentions in Current and Future Assisted Reproduction[1]

In the previous chapters, I discussed procreative responsibility, focusing primarily on the *consequences* of the future parent's actions and omissions. I argued that evaluating the consequences of a prospective parent's procreative choices, if limited to the person-affecting approach, allows for a reflection that can be considered appropriate by people embracing different moral theories.

However, although many agree that consequences are an essential aspect of morality, they may not be the only ones. For instance, several authors maintain that attitudes and intentions are also crucial aspects of morality, and considering them may be a helpful strategy to deal with procreative duties in order to overcome some of the counterintuitive implications of the consequences-based person-affecting morality (Bramble, 2021; Chambers, 2019; Kahane, 2009; Lotz, 2011; McDougall, 2007; Noggle, 2019; Wasserman, 2005). From this perspective, focusing on *why* parents want to make a specific procreative decision and, accordingly, on their intentions and attitudes may add pivotal details to our moral understanding of reproduction, giving us more tools for understanding our procreative duties.

Therefore, in this chapter, I focus on the role of procreative intentions and attitudes in defining procreative responsibility. More specifically, I aim to assess whether – and if so, how – attitudes and intentions can play a moral role in defining our *prima facie* moral duties regarding the use of Assisted Reproductive Technologies (ARTs) already available and those that may be available in the future, such as reproductive Genome Editing (rGE) and ectogenesis. Note that I am not going to argue that intentions and attitudes are morally relevant. Here, I merely acknowledge that for many people, such aspects are crucial in defining the morality of an action or omission, and then, assuming their relevance in nonprocreative contexts, I assess their possible role in defining procreative obligations. Moreover, by focusing on procreative attitudes and intentions, I do not intend to discard the fundamental role of consequences in

DOI: 10.4324/9781032654683-8

the definition of procreative responsibility, but rather to contribute to shaping a more holistic account of procreative responsibility capable of including additional relevant aspects of common-sense morality. Because of this, I will try to propose a convincing account able to justify the moral relevance of attitudes and intentions in defining procreative duties in a way *compatible* with the person-affecting morality and which can be integrated with the consequences-based person-affecting conclusions of the previous chapters. To be considered compatible, and hence relevant to this moral evaluation, attitudes and intentions should be person-affecting, namely, directed toward an actual person. From this perspective, positive and negative attitudes toward, say, creating a world with greater well-being than another (but without regard to the well-being of particular persons) should not be considered person-affecting any more than having positive or negative attitudes toward imaginary entities such as elves and goblins would be.

In line with the purposes of this book, I limit my investigation to procreative choices within the realm of ARTs. However, it is important to acknowledge that intentions and attitudes could also play a significant role in reproductive decisions that do not involve these technologies. Such choices include deciding to have a child under varying economic, social, or personal conditions. These aspects, though outside the scope of this book, warrant a deeper and more complex reflection and should be addressed in a different context. Nevertheless, the intentions, motivations, and attitudes of future parents in the context of ARTs, which appear more transparent and accessible for moral analysis according to David Wasserman (2005), provide a valuable starting point for a more comprehensive account.

This chapter is structured as follows. In Section 7.1, I will present and criticize one of the most influential accounts that consider attitudes and intentions to define procreative obligations in the field of genetic selection via Preimplantation Genetic Diagnosis (PGD), namely, the parental virtue approach. Then, in Subsection 7.1.1, I will criticize this model, arguing that, among other things, it provides no reason to claim that the virtuous procreator should pursue the same virtues as the parent. In light of this, in Section 7.2, I will consider two accounts proposed in the literature to justify the moral relevance of parental attitudes and motivations even in the procreative context. To overcome some of the criticisms encountered, in Section 7.3, I will propose the Parent–Child Relationship argument, which is based on the moral distinction between the intention to *create* and the intention to *parent* a child. I will argue that this argument offers a convincing way to deal with attitudes and intentions in a way compatible with person-affecting morality. Then, I will assess the implication of such an approach concerning the selective context, and I argue that some procreative choices involving PGD may be morally problematic – although they do not directly harm anyone – and this allows us to argue in favor of an extension of our procreative duties beyond what was prescribed by the consequences-based person-affecting morality. In Section 7.4, I will focus on procreative choices assuming that rGE and complete ectogenesis are available. I will first apply the Parent–Child Relationship argument in the field of rGE and argue that, in these circumstances, deciding to use *In Vitro* Fertilization (IVF) to put the future child in a position to be modified may even enhance the parent–child relationship, showing greater propensity by parents to take care of their child. I will claim that the same argument can be even better applied to ectogenesis. Then I will argue that if we consider procreative intentions and attitudes as morally relevant in these future scenarios, we may have moral reasons to prefer reproduction through these technologies rather than traditional reproduction. In this manner, the Bold Restriction of Procreative Autonomy model presented above will be rehabilitated, albeit with a limited normative force. This model was previously set aside in Chapter 4 (Subsection 4.4.1), where I focused solely on the moral relevance of consequences. Finally, in Section 7.5, I will return to the account discussed in the first part of this chapter, concluding that even for them the future availability of rGE and ectogenesis will determine additional moral constraints for prospective parents.

7.1   The Parental Virtue Approach

One of the most influential procreative responsibility models dealing with attitudes and intentions is the parental virtue approach. This normative perspective appears helpful for framing our reflection, as dispositions and character traits – central aspects of virtue ethics – inform and determine the intentions of agents. Although the appeal to virtue ethics in the procreative context has been proposed, more or less explicitly, by various authors,[2] in this section, I intend to discuss primarily the model proposed by Rosalind McDougall (2005, 2007, 2009). This model shares common features with other frameworks, including the call for unconditional love and acceptance of the future child; nevertheless, it advocates a relatively more permissive approach to ARTs, albeit still limited compared to what proponents of the Minimal Threshold Model (MTM) argue.

McDougall builds her proposal on the three premises of neo-Aristotelian ethics regarding the right action, developed by Rosalind Hursthouse (2001): (a) the criterion of the right action, according to which an action is right if and only if it is what a virtuous person would do in certain circumstances; (b) the nature of the virtuous person, which holds that a virtuous person is one who possesses and exercises virtues; and (c) the nature of virtues, which views virtues as traits that lead to human flourishing, taking the facts of human life as given.

From this perspective, unlike other normative theories, the concept of the virtuous person is primary and functional to that of the right action. Indeed, the virtuous person is one who possesses and exercises virtues, not one who follows certain normative rules. Hence, this approach asserts that virtues are traits a human being needs for *eudaimonia* or to flourish and live well. Virtue ethics is based on facts, such as certain tendencies or emotions, which are necessary to lead humans, as such, toward flourishing, like loyalty, justice, and kindness (Foot, 2001; Hursthouse, 1987). Nevertheless, basing virtues on the facts of human life does not commit the neo-Aristotelian to claim that virtuous humans inevitably flourish; rather, virtue is the only reliable bet in the pursuit of a good human life.

In light of this theoretical framework, McDougall applies the three premises of classic neo-Aristotelianism to the specific parental context, which are:

1 The Criterion of Right Parental Action: An action is right if and only if it is what a virtuous parent would do in the circumstances.
2 The Nature of the Virtuous Parent Claim: A virtuous parent is one who has and exercises the parental virtues.
3 The Nature of the Parental Virtues Claim: Parental virtues are character traits conducive to the flourishing of the child, taking facts about human reproduction as given (McDougall, 2007, p. 184).

According to McDougall, parental decisions begin before the child's existence and not only before birth but also before conception; in other words, they start when the parenting project is imminent. Therefore, some constraints that are proper for parents should apply to the procreative sphere. From these three premises, McDougall proposes three parental virtues that are particularly suitable for the procreative context, namely, *acceptingness, committedness*, and *future-agent-focus*. These virtues concur in favoring the flourishing of the future child, the primary and general aim of the virtuous parent.

Acceptingness is a virtuous parental trait since the child's characteristics will be unpredictable. Even knowing the entire genetic heritage of the future individual, the complexity of the environment in which it will be placed makes it impossible to know the totality of its phenotypic traits. Moreover, accepting the child regardless of their traits is commonly perceived as a necessary characteristic of the virtuous parent (Anderson, 1990; Cannold, 2003). John Robertson – an already mentioned proponent of a model compatible with MTM, which implies that individuals "deaf, hearing, 'ugly', dyslexic, short, tall, highly intelligent, etc." (Bennett, 2009, p. 271) can be selected – states that parents who use ARTs should still be committed to loving their child regardless of the outcome sought (Robertson, 2004).

The second virtuous trait corresponds to parental commitment: humans are born with physical and psychological needs that they cannot satisfy independently; therefore, they are in a situation of extreme dependence for which the parent must take responsibility.

Third, a virtuous parent should also preserve and, at the same time, promote the child's future autonomy, as a moral agent. This virtue is somehow compatible with the demands of the Child's Right to an Open Future argument, which has been discussed regarding genetic enhancement in Chapter 6.

Notice that such virtues should guide parenting choices while keeping in mind the Aristotelian idea of the golden mean. If a lack of acceptance reveals the vicious character of the parent, the same can be said of the propensity to accept any trait of the future individual. For example, passively accepting that a child develops aggressive character traits may not be what the virtuous parent should do.[3]

In light of this account, McDougall argues that parents-to-be should not seek specific traits such as the sex of their future child or aesthetic traits through selective reproduction since it would be contrary to acceptingness (McDougall, 2005). Embryo selection would be in line with acceptingness only if procreators tried to avoid a trait incompatible with the individual's flourishing, such as selecting against some quite severe disabilities.

A more controversial case is represented by the selection of certain traits that are generally considered as disabilities. Recall the case of Sharon Duchesneau and Candy McCullough, a couple who sought to have a deaf child using the sperm of a man with five generations of deaf relatives. The couple's choice to have a deaf child was motivated not so much by the intention of limiting the possibilities of the future individual but by the idea of having a child who would flourish within the context of a particular cultural identity. From this perspective, those parents seem in line with the virtue of commitment to the parenting project. McDougall claims, however, that some doubts may arise regarding the accordance with acceptingness. By seeking deafness in their future child, prospective parents would not accept the ability to hear, which certainly is not in contrast with the flourishing of the individual, in the same way as the sexual trait. Furthermore, according to McDougall, selecting a deaf individual would still contradict the virtue of future-agent-focus. Nevertheless, she also acknowledges that the latter could perhaps be construed as supporting the selection of a deaf child if they were raised within a deaf community (McDougall, 2009).

7.1.1 Criticisms of the Parental Virtue Approach

The parental virtue approach faces several criticisms. First, there is an objective difficulty in defining human flourishing, and McDougall's account may imply a very low requirement concerning the quality of life. Although she maintains that the intuitive concept of human flourishing requires a quality of life "far higher than the life-worth-living level" (McDougall, 2009, p. 356) and that the very concept of flourishing is not compatible "with the low threshold implied by the exclusively harm focused approach" (McDougall, 2005, p. 603), her proposal seems to go in the opposite direction. In this respect, Clara Saenz points out that McDougall offers an account that does not do justice to virtue ethics. While virtues, according to Saenz, should strive for excellence, McDougall seems to propose a minimum requirement in some ways comparable to that prescribed by MTM (Saenz, 2010). Indeed, we should notice that very few things can actually prevent a child from flourishing. Children, and humans in general, can flourish in very adverse circumstances: media often report stories of children who flourish despite serious health problems, poor family support, extreme poverty, etc. (Saenz, 2010). If acceptingness requires only that, through PGD, traits incompatible with flourishing be avoided, this seems to imply a rather minimal standard.

To this criticism, McDougall could reply that acceptingness is only one of the virtues to be considered: some traits may be compatible with it, but, at the same time, do not favor the promotion of the open future. However, this highlights a second problem with McDougall's model, namely, the inability to adequately inform procreative choices: shifting attention from one particular virtue to another reveals different and even incompatible duties involved in their child's flourishing, and this risks not providing future parents with a practical guide for procreative choices (Chambers, 2016).

Third – and more important for this chapter – we should note that selecting an embryo with a particular trait does not necessarily mean contradicting acceptingness, since the future parent could still welcome and accept the individual who will be born, regardless of their genetic characteristics, even if previously there was a selective process (Wilkinson, 2010). In other words, McDougall fails to acknowledge a substantial moral difference between preferring and attempting to create a child with specific characteristics and being disposed to reject a future child if they fail to have those characteristics. Let us assume that a couple wants to select an embryo that will develop into an individual who will have blue eyes and that, if this does not happen, the parents will give them up for adoption. Although it is clear that these parents are not guided by acceptingness, according to Stephen Wilkinson, this is not because they intend to select a child with specific characteristics (Wilkinson, 2010). Rather, it is due to their intention to reject the child if they have traits that differ from those they have selected for. Therefore, it is not unreasonable to argue that a reproducer can select an embryo with some specific characteristics and, subsequently, recognize that, since they decide to transfer it into the uterus, they will have to be guided by acceptingness and unconditional love.

This effective critique of acceptingness is based on the fact that it is not obvious that the procreators and parents encounter, at least in selective contexts, similar moral obligations. Since the future person does not yet exist, there may be reasons to claim that a procreator may have different obligations than the ones faced by a parent once the child exists. On the contrary, according to McDougall, procreators and parents should share the same moral attitudes informing their conduct; however, she does not provide any arguments to support this view, and this is one of the main reasons why McDougall's account seems unsatisfactory. Why should a procreator have specific attitudes or intentions toward a future child whose identity depends on those same attitudes and intentions that inform reproductive decisions? McDougall's account provides no clear answer to this question.

Although we may agree that parental character traits are morally relevant in a nonprocreative context, they are directed toward a specific individual whose identity does not depend on having or not having those parental character traits. Having parental virtues in the procreative context, however, may lead to conceiving in another moment, giving birth to another child, or leading to a different embryo from those resulting from the IVF process. In other words, such procreative attitudes are directed toward no specific future child; hence, they cannot be considered person-affecting.

This is even more evident if we consider not only acceptingness but also the future-agent-focus virtue. It is difficult to prescribe to the procreators to act in accordance with such a virtue, namely, to act bearing in mind the need for the future child to have an open future, if the action informed by this virtue, in fact, determines not so much the opening of the child's future, but what child will come into the world. Again, the future-agent-focus virtue may be perfectly plausible in a parental, nonprocreative context; however, this is not enough to claim that it should also be applied to the procreative one.

In sum, the parental virtue account thus constructed is not compatible with a person-affecting framework and McDougall does not provide a compelling argument for why a procreator should follow the same virtues as the parent. Without it, no prescription proposed by her would be adequately justified.[4] Therefore, to understand whether parental intentions and attitudes really matter in defining procreative duties, we need to build a different account that provides a justification of the intuition according to which, in some circumstances, selecting one embryo instead of another would be wrong because this would contradict appropriate parental attitudes or intentions.

7.2   Justifying the Moral Relevance of Procreative Intentions: Two Proposals

Some attempts have been made to justify the claim that procreators should possess certain parental attitudes and intentions, a matter which remains unresolved in McDougall's virtue ethics model. In this section, I will present two proposals. To facilitate the discussion, consider a new thought experiment that exemplifies the procreative attitudes and intentions that both proposals consider morally problematic:

Tanja and Ricky are both healthy carriers of a genetic mutation, which can lead to recessive disease D that, while compatible with a life worth living, significantly compromises the physical and mental well-being of the child and considerably reduces the number of opportunities to realize their life plan. The couple is aware of the severity of the disease and the suffering it entails; nevertheless, Tanja and Ricky believe that only having a child under those conditions would allow them to live a meaningful parenthood. Thus, they decide to undergo IVF and, subsequently, PGD to select and transfer into the uterus an embryo that will develop into a person affected by D, which is not currently curable effectively.

Many people might frown upon this and complain that this, like others already discussed, is a nonsensical example, far from reality and, thus, useless to address. For them, it is obvious that Tanja and Ricky are acting in a morally reprehensible way. Even conceding that the couple's choice does not harm the future child, they would still agree that the parents' attitudes are selfish and inconsiderate and, therefore, wrong. There would be no need for philosophical reflection on this. I strongly disagree with this view: to address the more complex cases, like the already mentioned case of Sharon Duchesneau and Candy McCullough, we need to deal with seemingly trivial cases. Indeed, as we will see, even justifying the moral intuition that Tanja and Ricky have performed a morally problematic action is more complex than common sense is willing to accept.

7.2.1 *Making Obligations Impossible to Fulfill*

The first proposal is offered by Robert Noggle (2019). He argues that if we accept that a good parent must protect their child from disease D and if D is not curable effectively and safely after birth, then Tanja and Ricky have moral reasons not to select, through PGD, an individual with D, because in this way Tanja and Ricky would be making it impossible to respect a moral duty that, as parents, they have toward their child.

Noggle bases his argument on a reformulation of the so-called "indirect strategy" (Tooley, 1985; Woodward, 1986). If we accept the already mentioned Kantian principle that "ought implies can", then we should recognize that selecting an embryo that will develop into a person with D, when D is not curable, cannot imply a duty for Tanja and Ricky to cure D. However, according to Noggle, the couple's act remains morally wrong. To justify this position, he claims that moral obligations do not always derive from the interests of specific individuals; in some contexts, they are instead determined solely by the intentions and attitudes of the agent. In this regard, Noggle proposes the Principle of Deliberate Impossibility (PDI), according to which it is morally wrong for a person P to perform action A at time t1 if P expects that performing A at time t1 will make it impossible for P to fulfill a moral obligation M at time t2 (Noggle, 2019). Consider the following case:

> Due to limited classroom space, the faculty in Pete's department take turns teaching a class during the dreaded 8:00 a.m. slot. Next semester, it is Pete's turn. The only practical way for Pete to get to campus by 8:00 a.m. is by driving. Knowing all this, Pete gives away his car and then announces that he cannot be obligated to teach the 8:00 a.m. class he has been assigned, since it is now impossible for him to get to campus that early.
>
> (Noggle, 2019, p. 2377)

According to PDI, Pete commits a morally problematic action because he attempts to escape a duty expected to be in force in the future, making himself incapable of fulfilling it. Similarly, since when the child is born they will have a duty to protect an actual person from D, Tanja and Ricky should not select an embryo with certain characteristics because, otherwise, it would not be possible to fulfill their moral obligation to protect the child from D. According to Noggle, failing to respect this moral duty is a moral evil, but an evil for which no one can complain, namely, *a non-grievance evil* (Feinberg, 1980), because it embodies defective attitudes and intentions, rather than harm toward an actual individual.

At this point, we should understand toward whom or what these defective attitudes and intentions are directed. PDI is conceived as a second-order obligation,[5] that is, an obligation that is not about harm to specific individuals but is primarily directed at one's first-order obligations, which in turn are intended toward other people (Noggle, 2019). While first-order obligations provide guidance on how we should behave toward a particular person, second-order obligations under the PDI indicate how to act regarding our first-order moral obligations. Therefore, the intention to violate this principle embodies a defective attitude not so much toward specific people, but toward moral norms themselves. Acting to avoid moral obligations in the future embodies contempt for morality itself. Such contempt is a negative characteristic of an action that is independent, or free-floating, from any wrong that might have been done to a specific individual toward whom an obligation, now impossible, would have been due.

Although it may seem strange to discuss an intention or attitude toward the moral obligation itself without it being directed toward a particular person, according to Noggle, this is quite familiar. Consider, for example, the canonical Kantian case where a person who despises their aunt recognizes a moral duty to visit her: in this context, the person embodies an appropriate attitude toward the moral obligation as such, even if they fail to embody an appropriate attitude toward their aunt (Noggle, 2019).

According to Noggle, this argument provides good reasons to support the view that Tanja and Ricky should not act with the awareness of putting themselves in a condition of being unable to fulfill a moral obligation. Therefore, couples intending to select an embryo with a disabling trait might encounter moral reasons not to do so. Note that this applies not only to couples who have an alternative to selecting an embryo with D (e.g., selecting another embryo) but also to couples who cannot and will never be able to conceive a child who is not affected by D. According to David Boonin, this last implication represents a strong criticism of Noggle's proposal, which would have created implausible implications than those it aims to avoid (Boonin, 2020).

Furthermore, in line with Boonin, I acknowledge that the moral duty to protect an individual from D might be overridden by the fact that this condition is necessary for their existence (Boonin, 2020). In the case of Tanja and Ricky, it is clear that D represents the necessary condition for the existence of the future individual; therefore, from this perspective, the duty to protect the child from D would cease to exist.

Finally, It is not entirely clear whether appealing to second-order reasons can justify a moral duty since it is not actually directed toward anyone, except toward the moral law itself. The same example proposed by Noggle can be understood in person-affecting terms since Pete shows attitudes toward actual people, Pete's colleagues, or Pete's future students, while this is not the case in the example of Tanja and Ricky. Even the Kantian example does not seem to fully help Noggle's argument. The positive attitude is indeed toward the moral law, which requires the individual to visit their aunt. But the Kantian moral law is a tool that brings out duties toward others, in this case, the aunt or toward oneself[6]; it certainly seems more difficult to consider a duty solely toward the moral law and, in general, a duty in the procreative context because this would seem not to be directed toward any specific individual.[7]

7.2.2 Procreative Intentions and Collective Interests

Mianna Lotz proposes a different argument to justify the moral relevance of parental intentions and attitudes in the procreative context. Like Noggle, Lotz acknowledges that moral evil in the procreative context cannot be contested by anyone to express grievances; however, the root of the moral defect lies not in the transgression of the moral norm itself but in a wrong toward the community (Lotz, 2011): procreative intentions and attitudes are relevant since they are directed toward a class to which people belong and in which they can identify. Therefore, the moral evil produced by procreating with certain motivations is in the direction of a collective wrong, defined as the deprivation of a common interest, an interest that people have as members of a community.

The community Lotz refers to is the moral one, thereby emphasizing a universalist rather than communitarian spirit. Such collective interests are attributable to all communities of agents and moral subjects, regardless of their interests and goals. Thus, the weakening of these collective goods and interests constitutes a setback for collective well-being. Procreation is a social activity that includes care, love, and the upbringing of the new generation: a task not only for the parents but also the entire community. Procreative attitudes and motivations, indeed, deal with the good and the future of the community and the world.

Although generally implicit, promoting certain intentions and motivations in procreation and other practices contributes significantly to forming and maintaining social bonds, and thus, "it contributes to the good and welfare of the moral community itself" (Lotz, 2011, p. 113). Therefore, Lotz suggests that all moral communities have, among their collective interests, an interest in individual procreative practices undertaken with the proper intentions and attitudes.

Procreation without adequate community consideration transgresses important collective ideals and interests; it fails to embody the moral community's self-evaluation. This establishes the community's legitimate interest in individual procreation, both in actual procreative conduct and in the attitudes, intentions, reasons, and motivations with which a new individual is generated. Lotz not only acknowledges the existence of a collective interest of the community in giving birth to its members without avoidable disabilities that are incompatible with or pose significant obstacles to achieving a decent quality of life, but goes a step further: she argues that there is a moral community interest even in the fact that its members do not intentionally generate children for purely ambitious or malign reasons, even where the children's lives exceed the minimum threshold of a life worth living.

Consider again the case of Tanja and Ricky. We can certainly argue that the couple's attitude contrasts with the collective interests discussed by Lotz. Nonetheless, the wrong toward the community would still be perpetrated even if the couple's child turned out not to be affected by the disability due to D. Regardless of its outcome, Tanja and Ricky's procreative action would still embody indifference toward suffering and, therefore, toward the moral community. However, the practical implications of Lotz's argument are more nuanced in other procreative contexts, as most procreative reasons and intentions will not be in direct or open conflict with the idea of contributing to the construction and replenishment of the moral community. From this perspective, it is not entirely clear whether procreative choices like those of Sharon Duchesneau and Candy McCullough are in contrast with the collective interests suggested by Lotz.

In general, Lotz wants to bring about a paradigm shift regarding reproduction, which is understood not only as a private practice but also, and especially, as a social one. In light of this consideration, we may acknowledge that Lotz's perspective considers procreative intentions and motivations not so much from a procreative-parental perspective, but from a reproductive one.

This paradigm shift is quite radical, as it not only considers the consequences of reproductive acts but also the underlying intentions. This approach can be perceived as a rather strong intrusion of the community's morality into the individual's private sphere. Intuitions and attitudes are socially less intelligible compared to the consequences of actions. This makes them less "manageable" and reliable within the framework of social morality. The socialization of procreative intentions might legitimize moralistic attitudes by the moral community on extremely personal, complex, and specific issues.

Conversely, as Lotz suggests, it is at least plausible to believe that reproductive attitudes and intentions can impact the collective welfare. This impact is understood in terms of how a moral community collectively perceives relevant values. When people show positive attitudes toward other people – and also toward other living beings – the moral community is strengthened, as reciprocal social expectations linked to promoting these positive attitudes are created, allowing for better coexistence. Parental attitudes certainly contribute to the well-being of the community in the terms described above. Similarly, the manifestation of certain parental attitudes in the procreative context can positively or negatively affect the moral community.

Note that this argument is immune from the already discussed criticism that the attitudes or intentions of parents and procreators would not be the same, and therefore, one could not ask the procreator to conform to certain parental attitudes. From the claim that public manifestation of parental attitudes in the procreative context is relevant to the well-being of the moral community, it does not follow that parental attitudes must be justified even in the procreative context. What is crucial is that the moral community *perceives* procreative attitudes as parental attitudes. Thus, if the moral community broadly views certain selective reproductive choices as detrimental – just *believing* that prospective parents would harm or wrong the future individual by displaying negative attitudes toward them – then expressing appropriate parental attitudes in reproductive contexts could enhance community welfare. Consequently, the moral community would benefit from encouraging specific parental attitudes among reproducers, even if these attitudes are not directly targeted at those seen as the recipients of parental care in the community's eyes.

Lotz's argument seems more plausible than Noggle's proposal and, unlike McDougall's, provides a justification for the importance of certain parental attitudes or virtues in the context of procreation. In the following section, however, I will present an alternative argument within the framework of procreative-parental responsibility based on the Parent–Child Relationship argument. This argument resists justifying the relevance of parental attitudes and intentions in the procreative context solely through community interests and concerns about reproductive responsibility.

7.3   The Parent–Child Relationship Argument

The Parent–Child Relationship argument has already been employed by several authors to define obligations in procreation. In Subsection 7.3.1, I start building the case for the Parent–Child Relationship argument by discussing and criticizing the existing accounts in the literature. Then, in Subsection 7.3.2, I propose a more refined version of the argument that can be adequately justified to assess procreative duties in assisted reproduction.

7.3.1   A First Definition

Anyone wishing to become a parent should acknowledge that through procreation, we bring about the creation not only of a new individual but also of a new relationship. Deciding to parent a child means creating a relationship that shapes the meaning of the lives of both the parent and the offspring (Chambers, 2019). This relationship is not only genetic but also psychological, physical, intellectual, and *moral*. According to Christine Overall, deciding to create a relationship means seeking a connection with a new human being, a connection that will not only bind the parent to that new human's needs but also make the parent themself needy and vulnerable in ways they have never been before (Overall, 2012). Although Overall argues that the fact of creating a "mutually enriching, mutually enhancing love that is the parent-child relationship" (Overall, 2012, p. 217)[8] provides the best moral reason for deciding to have a child, I do not have a position on this aspect; instead, I limit myself to observing that these considerations also make the parent–child relationship valuable in a certain way. The parent–child relationship is structurally asymmetrical since the parents decide not only to create a relationship but also to create the person with whom they will enter into a relationship. Furthermore, the child will initially be vulnerable, totally dependent, and needy. Without parents or other responsible adults, the child cannot survive. From this, it seems reasonable to claim that deciding to be in a parent–child relationship commits the parent to having some intention or attitude toward their child, namely, at the very least, a willingness to care for and protect them.

For the purposes of this chapter, it is crucial to assess whether the moral relevance of the parent–child relationship should also bind the procreator to the role of the parent and, therefore, have some parental attitudes and intentions. This does not seem so obvious considering that procreators and parents may reasonably have different roles and thus different obligations.

One argument in favor of this position is provided by K. Lindsey Chambers, who focuses on the moral relevance of the *beginning* of a relationship, which is as much a part of it as its midpoint or end. Because of this, procreators are committed to having at least some parental intentions and attitudes. Although people in a relationship may acquire greater or different obligations as the relationship progresses – such as when two people go from dating to becoming spouses – that does not mean there are no moral issues regarding how the relationship begins. She proposes a significant example, namely, a love affair. It implies that the partners admire and respect each other, not only once the relationship is in progress but also when it is about to begin. Starting a relationship inappropriately, such as pretending to engage in a sincere romantic relationship with someone with the express purpose of stealing from the partner and then draining their bank account, can corrupt the moral quality of the relationship, regardless of whether it subsequently gets better or worse. The scammer could sincerely fall in love with the partner they wanted to rob and decide not to pursue their primary purpose; however, this does not mean that the attitudes and intentions with which the love affair began are not morally blameworthy (Chambers, 2019). Likewise, Chambers argues, some procreative attitudes could reasonably corrupt the moral quality of the parent–child relationship.

What may be the implications of considering the relevance of the parent–child relationship in this way? The first answer may be that procreators should act with an attitude that contemplates the good of the future child with whom they will be in a relationship (Wasserman, 2005). At first glance, this may appear to be a rather demanding claim. If the decision to have a child must be motivated solely or primarily by the desire to give a good life to a future being, few parents could justify their procreative decisions, since many other reasons can drive people to procreate. From this perspective, parents-to-be who decide to have a child mainly because they would enrich the parents-to-be's existence or because this may repair their marriage could not "pass the test" of such a version of the Parent–Child Relationship argument.

However, in line with Wasserman, we can acknowledge that the good expected from the child's life can still play a significant role in decisions motivated in part by selfish reasons, preferences, attitudes, and intentions

(Wasserman, 2005). The desire to create and raise a child, or a specific kind of child, can be selfish in some respects, but this does not always exclude considerations related to the child's well-being and love for her. Therefore, even if parents cannot generate a child solely for reasons aimed at the child's own good, they could still create a child for reasons that *include* those aimed at the child's own good. In this "revised" version of the Parent–Child Relationship argument, morally problematic procreative choices are those informed *only* by selfish or sadistic intentions and attitudes.

Nevertheless, we should note that situations in which the prospective parent is not at all moved by certain attention to the good of the future individual are rare. Therefore, an appeal in these terms to the Parent–Child Relationship argument would produce rather weak moral constraints. For example, even Tanja and Ricky's choice to deliberately select a child with D could be considered morally appropriate, even though it is *mainly* (but not *solely*) motivated by selfish considerations. According to this version of the Parent–Child Relationship argument, if the prospective parents also have attitudes aimed at the well-being and care of their future child, their conduct is morally appropriate. I think that such an account of the argument requires too little. In the following subsection, I will claim that accepting the Parent–Child Relationship argument brings out greater procreative duties.

Moreover, it should be noticed that the Parent–Child Relationship argument understood in these terms may face serious criticisms that could potentially defeat it. Emphasizing the moral relevance of starting a new relationship to bind the procreator's conduct to the role of parent is not enough to speak of moral duties to act informed by certain intentions or attitudes in a procreative context: they would not be compatible with a person-affecting morality. Having different procreative attitudes and intentions may lead to conceiving at another moment in time, giving birth to a different child, or leading to a different embryo from those resulting from the IVF process. Although in a nonprocreative context, some attitudes and intentions may be relevant because they are directed toward a specific individual whose identity does not depend on having or not those parental character traits, this is not the case in the procreative context. In this respect, Chambers' example of the love affair is not suitable since it implies that the scammer has some negative attitudes toward an actual person, whereas it does not seem to be the case at the time of the decision to reproduce. Here, we can reasonably claim that the relationship is corrupted since the scammer did not respect an actual person at the beginning of their affair, regardless of whether the scammer later falls in love with the person he wanted to cheat and changes their mind about the scam; conversely, when prospective parents decide to procreate, they are not dealing with any actual person. In other words, the Parent–Child Relationship argument thus constructed encounters the same criticism faced by the parental virtue approach.

7.3.2 A More Refined Definition

I believe it is possible to provide a more convincing version of the Parent–Child Relationship argument, explaining why some parental attitudes and intentions are also morally relevant in the procreative context. To do this, we should appreciate a more sophisticated and morally relevant aspect emerging from the beginning of a parent–child relationship. This aspect also leads us to recognize that the parent–child relationship brings out greater moral demands than the minimum requirement of just considering the good of the future individual, and consequently, at least some procreative choices could be regarded as morally problematic, even though they do not harm the future child.

The beginning of a parent–child relationship in the context of an intentional procreative act implies two types of attitudes, namely, those that are purely reproductive and those that are genuinely parental. The former implies only wanting to *create* a child, while the latter implies wanting to *parent* one. Such a distinction is proposed by Guy Kahane – though he distinguishes between *creating* and *having* a child – who then derives, in the selective context, obligations like those that I also will accept in this and the following subsection (Kahane, 2009); however, he does not seem to link this distinction, at least directly, to the moral relevance of the parent–child relationship and its beginning. This generates problems in ultimately justifying the obligations he proposes. On the one hand, the distinction between *creating* and *parenting* a child enables us to justify the fact that the beginning of a parent–child relationship is also morally relevant in the procreative context, since – as I will argue in the following lines – it is possible to appreciate the existence of person-affecting attitudes in the decision to procreate. On the other hand, it should be noted that such a distinction by itself is not sufficient to state that procreators should be committed to having certain parental attitudes and intentions, since the justification of the moral constraints is still dependent on appreciating the moral value of the parent–child relationship and its beginning. By understanding this distinction through the lens of the Parent–Child Relationship argument, I believe that at least a further justification can be given for Kahane's conclusions.

To explain the moral relevance of the distinction between creating and parenting a child, let us consider again the example of Tanja and Ricky. Here, the procreators wish not only to create a child with D but also that any embryo chosen for transfer to the mother's womb develops into an individual with D. Although we often talk about "choosing an embryo with D" in the bioethical debate, this is inaccurate; according to Kahane, we should acknowledge that at the time of the embryo's creation, the latter is not literally affected by or free from D. An embryo at most has the biological potential to develop into a child free from D or affected by it. This is quite evident if we consider that the penetrance of many disease-causing mutations in a gene may not be complete, namely, when an embryo has a mutation that raises the risk of having a disease, but then the resulting child never develops it. Nevertheless, Kahane argues that even when we know for sure that the presence of a certain genetic variant determines that the child has disease D, e.g., an autosomal dominant mutation, it is not "metaphysically" impossible for the embryo to develop into an individual without D, namely, the future child could be different from how the prospective parents want it. This requires parents to implicitly formulate a second desire alongside that of creating a child with D; parents should also desire the embryo to develop into a child with D – which is the condition sought by the parents at the time of their creation – and that nothing happens, not even a "miracle" or the discovery of a cure for D, which prevents their future child from having D (Kahane, 2009).

Although the first desire, namely, creating a child with D, is not person-affecting since the identity of the child *directly depends* on the attitudes and intentions of the procreators, we should notice that the second desire or attitude is no longer aimed at an individual whose identity depends on the act informed by this desire; it is instead aimed at a specific individual. In other words, prospective parents would claim: "whatever embryo I will create and transfer to the uterus to have a child with D, I want that specific embryo to develop into a child with D".

Such a second desire is a sort of person-affecting one since it seems to be directed toward a specific person, even if, at the time of the parental decision, it is not yet known who that person will be. If we conceive this desire within the Parent–Child Relationship argument, we can observe that it can morally corrupt the relationship between the child and the parents, and it is precisely this that makes the prospective parents' choice to procreate with this desire morally problematic.

To clarify this point, consider the following example involving a relationship: Sally wants to have a roommate, so she puts an ad online. She does not know who the roommate will be, but whoever they are, she intends to lie to them about the rent, so that they will pay more than their fair share. Even though Sally does not know who her future roommate will be, her bad intention is still a person-affecting one. Clearly, Sally's actions harm the new roommate, who will be duped; nevertheless, and most importantly for the point discussed here, it is also a bad way to start the relationship that Sally will have with her roommate, whomever they are.

This problematic aspect seems independent of the occurrence or not of harm.[9] Even if the roommate turns out to be lovely and has a good relationship with Sally, who then changes her idea about duping them, or even if the scam will not harm the new flatmate but will benefit them overall (e.g., it could be that, even accounting for Sally's scam, the rent in this flat is significantly lower than that of comparable flats in the area), Sally has started the relationship in a morally problematic way. Tanja and Ricky, who intend for their future child (whoever that will be) to develop D, start their parent–child relationship in a similarly problematic way.

Note that this argument is not intended to support that the second desire should be understood in the *de dicto* rather than *de re* sense as discussed in Chapter 3. The second desire proposed here – namely, hoping and wanting that, whatever the identity of the future child will be, they will develop in order to have certain characteristics – refers to a specific person even if we do not yet know who that person will be. To put it in an example, let us consider again the case of Sally, who does not know the future flatmate she would like to scam; however, even though she does not know who her flatmate will be, by putting the ad online, she will start a relationship with them, who is a specific person, in a morally problematic way. In positive terms, let us consider the initiatives of adopting a child from a distance. When I decided to donate money to adopt this child, I did not know their identity, but I am still starting a relationship with the child that will be assigned to me by the charity organization.

In light of this, I argue that the Parent–Child Relationship argument commits procreators to having attitudes and intentions that are not in contrast with the desires and hopes that their children's lives go well and that they are safe from suffering. These requirements overcome the minimal ones proposed in the previous subsection, which only suggested considering the good of the future individual as one aspect of the procreative decision. If we acknowledge that through the procreative act, prospective parents also intend to parent a future child and not just create one, then it follows that they face moral reasons to act with some parental attitudes and intentions by virtue of the new relationship that they will necessarily create. In other words, in contrast with the minimum standard account discussed in the previous subsection, prospective parents would be required not only to have attitudes and intentions that include the good of the future individual but also to have attitudes and intentions that are not in conflict with those expected to guide parents once the child is born.

Notice that the fact that the future child's identity depends on the parents' actions – and consequently also on their intentions and attitudes – does not exempt Tanja and Ricky from having moral reasons to consider a genetic disease like D as undesirable for the child, namely, an individual with whom parents will enter a relationship that obliges them to maintain certain attitudes toward the child. The moral relevance of the parent–child relationship commits prospective parents to desire and hope that their children's lives go well and that they are safe from harm. This is the same constraint that, according to many people, parents of an already existing child encounter.

Of course, the moral defect of the second desire discussed here cannot be considered an actual "harm" to the future individual. The fact that pro-creators have sadistic and exclusively selfish impulses does not necessarily make the life of their future child better or worse, as long as it is worth living, since the alternative is non-existence. Nonetheless, I argue that, re-gardless of the considerations linked to the harm toward the future indi-vidual, it is still possible to *wrong* them. The individual born thanks to the sadistic and selfish impulses of the parent cannot complain of being born in the only condition in which they can exist; however, they may still be sorry or resentful that the parent has started the parent–child relationship with conduct informed by an attitude that is contrary to parental attitudes of care. What is corrupted through some procreative choices is, in fact, the parent–child relationship at its very beginning.

Notice that this argument is not committed to claiming that *all* the par-ents' attitudes or desires must necessarily be in line with loving or protect-ing them, but only the desires and attitudes that inform their conduct.[10] A parent may feel envy or have the desire to wrong the child for many reasons or to prevent them from leaving the family house or country to pursue a great career for the sake of enjoying a greater closeness with them. However, as long as the parent perceives those desires as out of line with "proper parenting" and then decides to act informed by other attitudes and intentions that align with childcare, they do not undermine the parent–child relationship and cannot be considered a "bad parent". Often, we are not in control of our desires and attitudes, and prescribing people to have specific desires and attitudes even if they do not inform our conduct seems like an overly moralistic intrusion into the human psyche. What we can do, however, is critically reflect on our desires and, hence, act appropriately by deciding which desires should inform our conduct. In this way, the Parent–Child Relationship argument proposed here can maintain that desires and attitudes are important to moral conduct without embracing overly implau-sible assumptions about the moral relevance of attitudes and intuitions, for example, that *all* our desires should be committed to love and care of the child even though they do not ultimately inform parents' conduct.

The Parent–Child Relationship argument thus constructed presents at least two advantages over the parental virtue approach, PDI, and the pre-vious version of the Parent–Child Relationship argument. First, thanks to the distinction between creating and parenting a child, it can under-lie attitudes and intentions compatible with the person-affecting morality, avoiding criticism faced by the other approaches. Second, it does not need to rely directly on some specific normative account, such as virtue ethics or some specific kind of deontology. This argument only assumes an intuition that many people share – and that several moral theories could defend – that some specific intentions and attitudes, such as caring, should inform parents' conduct; accordingly, actions or omissions informed by intentions and attitudes in conflict with "proper parenthood" should be considered morally problematic. If we accept this and recognize the plausibility of the Parent–Child Relationship argument that I proposed in this section, we should be committed to accepting the conclusions that we discuss in the next sections.

7.3.3 Implications of the Parent–Child Relationship Argument in the Selective Context

The Parent–Child Relationship argument has relevant implications for procreative-parental responsibility in the selective context. Procreators moved by sadistic and selfish attitudes – who use IVF plus PGD to intentionally select an embryo with certain characteristics that favor the aims of domination and control over the future child – would not start the parent–child relationship in a morally appropriate way. They not only intend to create an individual under certain conditions but also prefer that the child develop certain conditions, and this would give the child reasons for resentment. Even if she could not have existed otherwise, she can point out a moral defect in the attitudes that led to the beginning of the relationship she has with her parents. The relationship started in a bad way because of the moral attitude of the parents, who desired and hoped that the child would develop a condition involving suffering or disability. Although this condition is necessary for the existence of the future child, this does not legitimize the prospective parents demonstrating indifference to or even taking satisfaction in the fact that the child experiences such suffering.

From this perspective, not only sadistic and selfish parents but also future parents with a disability who want a child similar to themselves – but at the same time recognize this condition is likely to cause suffering or reduce opportunities – can be at odds with the Parent–Child Relationship argument (Kahane, 2009).

Nevertheless, there are cases in which the desire to create a child under certain conditions is not in line with the desire for them to develop under the same conditions. Consider a couple who discovers after IVF plus PGD that they can only have a child with disease D. On the contrary to Tanja and Ricky, in this case, the couple does not necessarily want the child to develop D. They could decide to proceed with the parenting project without showing indifference toward the condition that their child will experience. In this context, the parents' relationship with their future child is by no means incompatible with the desire for love and care. Therefore, they do not display any defective or vicious attitudes or intentions.

Likewise, according to the Parent–Child Relationship argument, there is no ground for criticizing future parents who leave it to chance to decide which child they will have. In this case, the parents do not intend to create an individual with D or necessarily parent an individual with D.

Moreover, there may be cases in which parents with a desire to parent a child with D conceive D as a trait causing neither disability nor suffering. Consider again the case of Sharon Duchesneau and Candy McCullough; in this context, the parents did want the embryo to develop into a deaf child, but according to the couple, deafness is neither a trait that significantly compromises the physical and mental well-being of the child nor does it significantly reduce the number of opportunities for those affected to implement their life plans.[11]

Someone may argue that although the intentions and attitudes considered in themselves are not subject to moral blame, they are misinformed. That is, the desire for the child to develop into a condition that does not lead to disability is incompatible with the action of selecting an embryo that will develop in an individual with deafness since this condition cannot fail to be a disability. If this were true, then the intention of the couple would be morally legitimate but it would be incompatible with the action informed by it (Kahane, 2009). Here, we notice again that procreative responsibility strictly depends on what definition of disability we consider appropriate. In Chapter 2, I have already discussed the concept of disability, discussing the Welfarist and Equal Opportunities models; in this regard, I acknowledged that these models provide good reasons to *generally* consider deafness as a disability. If this were true, then the couple's intention would be morally legitimate in itself; however, it would be incompatible with the action informed by it. The moral blame would fall not so much on the intention, but on the fact that the latter could be compatible with the parents' action. However, in line with many authors, we note that if one does not consider D or deafness as a disability, then one should be committed to claiming that, in some cases, it is morally legitimate to *cause* D or deafness in an existing individual (Brock, 2005; Kahane, 2009; McMahan, 2005).

The argument that I support here fails to justify the intuition according to which it would be morally problematic to generate a life barely worth living without, however, hoping that this life will develop and then remain in that situation. Consider a couple who discovers after IVF plus PGD that they can only have a child in a much more serious condition than existence with D, but, in any case, has a life that is barely worth living. Many people would agree that prospective parents are behaving in a morally wrong way if they decide to become pregnant, even if the life of their future child would be minimally worth living. There seem to be no reasons to support the moral wrongness of this conduct, as long as this is also motivated by parental love for creating a new relationship and not by the selfish or sadistic desire that this trait remains in the future individual. However, a prudential argument could be advanced: since it is highly probable that a life just worth living could become unsustainable, this would offer a reason to avoid procreating such a life even if this is not necessarily contrary to the possibility that the generated individual has a life worth living (Glover, 2006).

Finally, in terms of the selection of non-health-related traits, such as sex or eye color, the Parent–Child Relationship argument does not seem to conflict with the attitudes and intentions that inform procreative actions in this area. Choosing to have a child with blue or brown eyes or of a specific sex does not seem contrary to an attitude of care and protection toward the child: the future parent does not want the child to develop a suffering condition or disability, but in a nonharmful condition that falls within the range of normal functioning of human beings that meets the parent's preferences. Therefore, there is good reason to believe that such intentions are not necessarily morally problematic, though they would be so if the parent decided to give the child up for adoption if the latter did not present the desired character. The second desire involved in this type of decision is similar to that of a couple who hopes that their future child will be male or female or of another couple who instead hopes that their child has blue eyes. These wishes appear to align with or at least not conflict with care and protection for the future child. This aspect also allows us to appreciate a further difference with the parental virtue approach.

In sum, the Parent–Child Relationship argument allows us to state that, in the selective context, at least some procreative intentions and attitudes are morally problematic in a way compatible with person-affecting morality, even if no one is harmed by the parent-to-be's behavior. Therefore, we can acknowledge that even in the selective context procreators encounter greater moral constraints than those proposed by MTM, according to which all procreative choices are legitimate except for giving birth to a child with a life not worth living.

7.4 Applying the Parent–Child Relationship Argument to Future Scenarios: Toward a Revision of the Greater Moral Obligation View?

Let us apply the Parent–Child Relationship argument to a scenario in which future and still hypothetical reproductive techniques such as rGE and ectogenesis are available. Let us first consider rGE. To understand the moral role of attitudes and intentions in the field of rGE, remember that in previous chapters I argued that rGE is a non-identity-affecting technique. In light of this, in Chapter 4 (Section 4.3), I argued that parents who already are in the IVF process, namely, when the numerical identity of the future children already exists, have moral duties not to harm the future individual by using or refraining from using rGE, based on consequences-based person-affecting morality. Considering attitudes and intentions, failing to respect such moral obligation should be morally wrong not only because it harms the future person, but also because such conduct would imply procreative attitudes contrary to the parent–child relationship, namely, the parental role that the procreator plays in that moment. Note, however, that here I am considering the moral relevance of procreative intentions when the prospective parents are already in the IVF process, namely, in a post-conception scenario. This certainly makes it easier to justify that parents are required to have some parental attitudes toward the person who will surely exist since there is someone toward whom parents' intentions and attitudes are directed, namely, the future child. Nevertheless, appealing to attitudes and intentions may be redundant if we already recognize and accept the existence of some consequences-based person-affecting obligations.

Assessing whether intentions and attitudes play a role in informing procreative decisions is more relevant in pre-conception scenarios, namely, when the embryo numerically identically to the future person does not yet exist. In this context, consequences-based person-affecting morality cannot inform prospective parents' conduct, since, at the time of this decision, the embryo sharing the same numerical identity with the future child does not yet exist. Instead, I argue that if we accept the Parent–Child Relationship argument, we should be committed to supporting the existence of new moral duties even in the pre-conception scenario.

To demonstrate this, we should note that assuming that rGE is a non-identity-affecting procedure also implies that the availability of such a procedure allows us to increase control over the life of whoever will be our child when the latter is procreated via IVF. While through natural reproduction there is limited control over some characteristics of the future person, the implementation of rGE would allow an extension of the parent's power, since the embryo could be qualitatively modified before being transferred to the mother's womb. By deciding to reproduce through IVF in light of the availability of rGE, prospective parents put whoever will be their future child in a condition in which she can be affected – either benefited or harmed – more by the parents' decisions than a child created via natural reproduction.[12] Therefore, by having a future child who can be affected more by their decisions, prospective parents would have more opportunities to express their parenting attitudes and intentions toward the future individual, namely, more room to express care and protection toward their future child.

Consider again the two desires implied in creating a new parent–child relationship and apply them to rGE. As in the selective context, the future parents are committed to having two distinct desires when they decide whether to procreate through IVF in light of the availability of rGE. The first is to create one or more embryos: such a desire is immune from moral praise or blame because it is not addressed to any specific individual. Here, our desires, attitudes, and intentions cannot find a personal target toward whom to be directed. The second desire, implicit in the prospective parents' decision, may instead be that, whatever the identity of the embryo, it can develop in the ideal conditions to prevent the future child from being harmed or suffering. This second desire has a specific individual as a target, that is, any embryo that will be created by the IVF process and will be subjected to rGE or not, even if, at the time of formulating the desires, the parents do not yet know the identity of their child.[13]

Such a desire not only undermines the parent–child relationship but even enhances and promotes it: as a matter of fact, given the availability of rGE, the parents' decision to resort to IVF can be understood as an action aimed at increasing control over the well-being and opportunities of the future child, thus demonstrating a greater propensity to take care of the interests of their child during the beginning of the parent–child relationship. Through the decision to reproduce with IVF, prospective parents deliberately decide to bring into the realm of procreative responsibility the characteristics of the future child that can be affected by rGE – characteristics that would not have been alterable through sexual intercourse. The prospective parents take charge of the initial step of the development of the future individual that, by opting for artificial reproduction, falls within the field of choice, and therefore of morality, and no longer of chance. Thus, if we accept the plausibility of the Parent–Child Relationship argument, then the availability of rGE leads us to have moral reasons for preferring reproduction through IVF to natural reproduction.[14] Such a choice allows us to enhance the parental attitudes of care and protection toward the future child, and it would be the best way to begin the parent–child relationship. This is no longer a neutral choice, as for the consequence-based person-affecting morality, but a morally relevant one.

This argument is somewhat morally similar to a more familiar one according to which a parent with a young child would have moral reasons to accept a job offer that guarantees them a better salary because, in this way, they could provide the child with more educational opportunities, better healthcare, and so forth. Again, thanks to a better wage, the parent can afford to take care of the child more compared to a scenario in which the parent had not accepted the job offer. The child certainly benefits from this choice in comparative terms, but the parent–child relationship is also improved as the parent shows a greater caring attitude toward the child.

Of course, in the rGE context, the child cannot be harmed or benefited by the parent's decision to employ IVF to use or not use rGE, since such decisions determine their existence and, consequently, their identity. However, the child may not only not feel regret at the parent's decision but even be pleased because this act embodied procreative intentions and attitudes aimed at protecting and caring for the child themself.

This line of thought does not apply only to rGE but also, and perhaps above all, to the future and still hypothetical possibility of complete ectogenesis. As already noted in Chapter 4 (Subsection 4.4.3), complete ectogenesis would allow taking care of the future child, from its very beginning until its birth. Deciding to procreate using it would be a decision that can embody morally positive attitudes toward the future individual, who is put in a position to be protected in a greater way than in a natural pregnancy.[15]

Some might argue that, as for rGE, the use of ectogenesis could be more easily justified based on consequences once we are in a post-conception scenario, that is, when the embryo is created. The already existing embryo would be in a condition to be harmed or benefited by the use or not of ectogenesis. However, some might even claim that the choice to transfer the embryo to the uterus rather than resorting to ectogenesis could promote a better relationship, through body sharing between the mother and the fetus, than ectogenesis.[16] I do not want to enter into this issue. Here, I limit myself to saying that in a pre-conception scenario, where no reasons based on consequences may apply, a parent encounters moral reasons for preferring to procreate through ectogenesis over natural reproduction.

In light of such considerations, I argue that considering attitudes and intentions in defining procreative responsibility through the lens of the parent–child relationship in the context of the aforementioned future scenarios leads us to rehabilitate, albeit with a different justification and a different normative claim, the Bold Restriction of Procreative Autonomy model, which should be reformulated as follows:

> All prospective parents in the economic and technological conditions to do so have moral reasons to reproduce through the following practices
>   (a) IVF, in such a way as to subject the designated embryo to transfer *in utero* to rGE every time the latter is affected by treatable genetic diseases that harm the future person;
>   (b) Ectogenesis, in such a way as to subject the developing embryo to treatments, genetic or otherwise, whenever the latter is affected by conditions potentially harmful to the future person.

This is justifiable not so much because of the potential harm inflicted on the future individual, but because of the parental intentions and attitudes of care and protection required of future parents in the procreative context. From this perspective, these reproductive technologies make it possible to enhance and promote the parent–child relationship more than natural reproduction. Applying the Parent–Child Relationship argument not only "reaffirms" the duties already established by the Mild Restriction of Procreative Autonomy regarding rGE for parents-to-be who are already in the IVF process but also justifies brand new significant moral reasons, further expanding procreative responsibility.

Again, for these moral constraints to be applied, the techniques under discussion must be effective, safe, legal, and economical. Moral reasons or duties based on intentions and attitudes are certainly less stringent than those based on consequences. Nevertheless, if we accept their moral relevance, these can at least play a role in informing our choices in the procreative context. Moreover, remember that such moral constraints should not be conceived as absolute but as *prima facie*; therefore, they must be weighed against other morally relevant issues in the reproductive context, such as psychological, physical, and social burdens or other morally relevant considerations.

A final remark is needed. It is important to note that in this section I confined the discussion of the Parent–Child Relationship argument to the avoidance of harmful conditions via non-identity-affecting procedures. Therefore, the implications of this argument for genetic enhancement in both pre-conception and post-conception scenarios were not addressed.[17] In other words, I have not explored whether the Parent–Child Relationship argument may provide moral reasons to forbid, allow, or require genetic enhancement. This choice stems from two reasons: first, in this chapter, as in Chapter 4, my primary interest was in understanding *when* moral reasons that can inform procreative choice arise, rather than delineating specific moral obligations. My aim was indeed to understand whether prospective parents have a *prima facie* moral duty to give up traditional reproduction in favor of using ARTs. Second, there is substantial disagreement about how moral positions based on the moral relevance of the parent–child relationship should engage with genetic enhancements. Some have expressed doubts about whether genetic enhancements could be considered legitimate, since it is very likely that they violate unconditional love or express some problematic attitudes of hyperparenting (Prusak, 2013; Sandel, 2009). Conversely, it might be argued that if such enhancements are promoted with the intention of increasing the opportunities of the future individual – in line with the Childs' Right to an Open Future argument – the parent–child relationship is not compromised at all, and they should be considered permissible. Ultimately, an appealing interpretation of the Parent–Child Relationship argument could even bring out new moral reasons to enhance future children since guaranteeing more opportunities through genetic enhancement to the future child would be a great expression of love toward children (Brock, 2009), even more than the attitudes of care and protection of children required by the Bold Restriction for Procreative Autonomy. Further reflection is needed to address this crucial issue. Here, my aim was more modest, and I believe that both sides of the debate could *at least* agree with the minimal conclusions I have put forward.

7.5 Returning to Previous Accounts

The argument in favor of the Bold Restriction of Procreative Autonomy is not defensible from a relational perspective alone; on the contrary, it seems to me that all other accounts dealing with attitudes and intentions presented in this chapter converge in supporting that the availability of rGE and ectogenesis, as procedures extending possible control over the traits of future children, raises moral reasons to prefer artificial reproduction over natural reproduction.

First, consider the parental virtue approach, according to which a virtuous parent should be informed by acceptingness, parental commitment, and future-agent-focus. Acceptingness may pose a *prima facie* obligation to refuse the use of ARTs, as this would contrast with unconditionally accepting the traits of the future individual. However, I believe that the availability of rGE or ectogenesis is not in conflict with such virtue, since a prospective parent intending to use one of these two techniques might want to place a particular person in a protected environment where they can value the parental commitment to care for the child from the earliest embryonic stages, regardless of the starting characteristics of the created embryo. Therefore, there would be moral reasons to choose to reproduce through such a practice, as it would promote the virtue of parental commitment without necessarily compromising that of acceptance. Note that the availability of rGE and ectogenesis would not inevitably make vicious the procreator who decides not to resort to them, although the procreator who places their future child in a condition to be protected thanks to them would probably be more virtuous.

Critics like Robert Sparrow might point out that rGE, at least in its early clinical applications, would still involve embryo selection either before or after modification (Sparrow, 2022), and this, again, would demonstrate a tendency in contrast with acceptingness. I have already argued that it is controversial to claim that the future parent demonstrates vicious behavior simply by selecting one embryo over another since the procreator could not assume a parental attitude even toward the merely possible individuals who could have been their children. Nevertheless, if we focus on the child who will exist rather than on the process that leads to their existence, we can still observe that the embryo from which the child developed was placed in conditions to be protected. This would enhance the virtue of parental commitment.

Regarding the account proposed by Noggle, we should recognize that deciding to employ rGE and ectogenesis does not make it impossible to comply with a second-order obligation, unlike some selective practices. On the contrary, the availability of such techniques would make it possible to extend parental control. If, in light of PDI, we recognize that it is morally problematic to act in a way that makes future obligations impossible to fulfill, it is also reasonable to argue that expanding the sphere of the moral duty of care and protection towards one's offspring is both good and desirable. This is because prospective parents would have more opportunities to fulfill their obligation toward the child and respect the moral law. Therefore, Noggle appears committed to arguing that rGE and ectogenesis expand procreative-parental responsibility and that there are moral reasons to resort to artificial reproduction rather than natural reproduction.

Finally, consider Lotz's proposal, according to which certain procreative attitudes conflict with collective interests. As I have argued, employing rGE and ectogenesis could embody procreative attitudes such as care towards the future individual in an unprecedented way, attitudes that were not present in the ordinary and selective procreative contexts. Acting in the procreative context motivated by the propensity for care and protection of the future individual could promote a greater collective interest connected to the well-being of the moral community. Therefore, valuing such motivations through the use of these reproductive techniques within the moral community to which one belongs would be morally desirable.

Notes

1 This chapter revisits and expands upon the work presented in Battisti (2023), frequently employing the same wording as the original published article.
2 See, for instance, Parens and Asch (2003) and Sandel (2009).
3 Note that McDougall is not clear whether this example refers to an individual who already exists or to the possibility of selecting or modifying the embryo to eliminate any potential aggressive disposition.
4 This argument is also helpful in responding to a possible objection to the criticism I have put forward regarding acceptingness. According to this objection, acceptingness should not be understood as a disposition toward someone, but rather as a stable trait of character that one either possesses or does not. From this perspective, one could not exhibit virtue only toward the embryo that is chosen and not toward the one that is discarded. Discarding an embryo because it does or does not possess certain traits is a sign of a general lack of virtue in the character of the procreator. However, as long as the thesis for which the acceptingness should also be extended toward merely possible people is not justified, it cannot be maintained that acceptance should also be directed

toward the embryo that is decided to be discarded. Therefore, there is a need for an argument that McDougall, however, does not provide.

5 In Battisti, Capulli, and Picozzi (forthcoming), I use the distinction between first- and second-order reasons differently. Nevertheless, here I follow what is suggested by Noggle.

6 From a Kantian perspective, it might be interesting to attempt to justify certain procreative duties as duties toward oneself, rather than toward the moral law as such; this operation has also been proposed concerning duties toward animals. For a discussion on this, see Camenzind (2021). Nonetheless, the most widespread opinion in the contemporary debate is that there are only duties toward others, while duties toward ourselves are controversial, if not outright "fraudulent concepts" (Williams, 1985, p. 185).

7 This is the reason why authors like Manninen argue that since Kantian ethics, especially through the second formulation of the categorical imperative, is based on respect for existing persons, it cannot solve the procreative dilemmas under discussion (Manninen, 2012). For a critique of this perspective, see Patrone (2017).

8 In a different vein, Weinberg (2015) argues that the desire to engage in the parent–child relationship is a valid and morally acceptable motivation that justifies procreation, which always involves imposing "life's risks" on children.

9 I am deeply indebted to Gary O'Brien, who suggested this example.

10 I thank Silvia Ceruti for discussion on this point.

11 This belief is in line with the Mere Difference View, according to which disability does not make a person overall worse off, but is just a difference, such as sexual orientation, the color of the skin, and gender. For a defense of this perspective, see Barnes (2016).

12 Of course, a pregnant person could affect the child before birth, say, taking teratogenic drugs, or doing something that could cause harm to the child. However, here, I just argue that if prospective parents decide to undergo IVF and rGE is available, they can potentially affect some characteristics of the future child in a way that is not possible in an embryo created via sexual intercourse.

13 Some couples or single reproducers may want to undergo IVF plus rGE in order to *cause* disability in the future child. This is still in contrast with the Parent–Child Relationship argument in the same way that it is for a couple that selects for disability in those circumstances I mentioned above.

14 This conclusion is not new. For example, it was proposed, among others, by Harris (1993). Nonetheless, the reasons I use to support this conclusion are different from those used by Harris.

15 Some might argue that ectogenesis requires a radical rethinking of the relationship between fetus and mother and this could have negative consequences on the parent–child relationship. Therefore, it should not be employed. For the sake of this argument, I argue that these moral reasons should be balanced as I suggest at the end of this section. Here, I just observe that moral reasons also emerge for deciding to reproduce via ectogenesis rather than natural reproduction.

16 I thank Massimo Reichlin for bringing out this point.

17 It should be remarked that I do not consider the use of genetic selection via PGD to select non-health-related traits as genetic enhancement, since in this context the embryo is selected because of the characteristics it already possesses. So, the claim that I did not address the case of genetic enhancement is perfectly consistent with the fact that I discussed the implications for the

Parent–Child Relationship argument for selection of some aesthetic traits in Subsection 7.3.3. Although it is possible that some considerations about the Parent–Child Relationship argument proposed in the context of genetic selection of non-health-related traits could also be applied to the context of genetic enhancement via non-identity-affecting practices, there may be differences that warrant further investigation, especially for those genetic enhancements that have a substantial impact on well-being and opportunities, compared to others such as changing eye or hair color.

References

Anderson, E. S. (1990). Is women's labor a commodity? *Philosophy & Public Affairs, 19*(1), 71–92.

Barnes, E. (2016). *The minority body: A theory of disability.* Oxford University Press.

Battisti, D. (2023). Attitudes, intentions and procreative responsibility in current and future assisted reproduction. *Bioethics, 37*(5), 449–461.

Battisti, D., Capulli, E., & Picozzi, M. (forthcoming). The first and second-order ethical reasons approach: The case of human challenge trials. *Ethics and Human Research.*

Boonin, D. (2020). Solving the non-identity problem: A reply to Gardner, Kumar, Malek, Mulgan, Roberts and Wasserman. *Law Ethics and Philosophy,* 127–156.

Bramble, B. (2021). The defective character solution to the non-identity problem. *The Journal of Philosophy, 118*(9), 504–520.

Brock, D. W. (2005). Shaping future children: Parental rights and societal interests. *The Journal of Political Philosophy, 13*(4), 377–398.

Brock, D. W. (2009). "Is selection of children wrong?" In J. Savulescu & N. Bostrom (Eds.), *Human enhancement* (pp. 251–276). Oxford University Press.

Camenzind, S. (2021). Kantian ethics and the animal turn. On the contemporary defence of Kant's indirect duty view. *Animals: An Open Access Journal from MDPI, 11*(2), 512.

Cannold, L. (2003). Do we need a normative account of the decision to parent? *The International Journal of Applied Philosophy, 17*(2), 277–290.

Chambers, K. L. (2016). *Choosing our children: Role obligations and the morality of reproductive selection.* University of California.

Chambers, K. L. (2019). Wronging future children. *Ergo (Ann Arbor, Mich.), 6*(20201214). https://doi.org/10.3998/ergo.12405314.0006.005

Feinberg, J. (1980). Legal moralism and freefloating evils. *Pacific Philosophical Quarterly, 61*(1–2), 122–155.

Foot, P. (2001). Practical rationality. In *Natural goodness* (pp. 52–65). Oxford University Press.

Glover, J. (2006). *Choosing children.* Oxford University Press.

Harris, J. (1993). *Wonderwoman and superman.* Oxford Paperbacks.

Hursthouse, R. (1987). *Beginning lives.* Blackwell.

Hursthouse, R. (2001). *On virtue ethics.* Oxford University Press.

Kahane, G. (2009). Non-identity, self-defeat, and attitudes to future children. *Philosophical Studies, 145*(2), 193–214.

Lotz, M. (2011). Rethinking procreation: Why it matters why we have children. *Journal of Applied Philosophy, 28*(2), 105–121.

Manninen, B. A. (2012). What did octomom do wrong? Exploring the ethics of fertility treatments. *APA Newsletter on Philosophy and Medicine, 12*(1), 11–14.

McDougall, R. (2005). Acting parentally: An argument against sex selection. *Journal of Medical Ethics, 31*(10), 601–605.

McDougall, R. (2007). Parental virtue: A new way of thinking about the morality of reproductive actions. *Bioethics, 21*(4), 181–190.

McDougall, R. (2009). Impairment, flourishing, and the moral nature of parenthood. In K. Brownlee & A. Cureton (Eds.), *Disability and disadvantage* (pp. 352–368). Oxford University Press.

McMahan, J. (2005). Causing disabled people to exist and causing people to be disabled. *Ethics, 116*(1), 77–99.

Noggle, R. (2019). Impossible obligations and the non-identity problem. *Philosophical Studies, 176*(9), 2371–2390.

Overall, C. (2012). *Why have children?* MIT Press.

Parens, E., & Asch, A. (2003). Disability rights critique of prenatal genetic testing: Reflections and recommendations. *Mental Retardation and Developmental Disabilities Research Reviews, 9*(1), 40–47.

Patrone, T. (2017). Kant's 'formula of humanity' and assisted reproductive technology: A case for duties to future children. *Monash Bioethics Review, 34*(3–4), 206–225.

Prusak, B. G. (2013). *Parental obligations and bioethics.* Routledge.

Robertson, J. A. (2004). Procreative liberty and harm to offspring in assisted reproduction. *American Journal of Law & Medicine, 30*(1), 7–40.

Saenz, C. (2010). Virtue ethics and the selection of children with impairments: A reply to Rosalind McDougall. *Bioethics, 24*(9), 499–506.

Sandel, M. J. (2009). *The case against perfection.* Belknap Press.

Sparrow, R. (2022). Human germline genome editing: On the nature of our reasons to genome edit. *The American Journal of Bioethics: AJOB, 22*(9), 4–15.

Tooley, M. (1985). *Abortion and infanticide.* Oxford University Press.

Wasserman, D. T. (2005). The nonidentity problem, disability, and the role morality of prospective parents. *Ethics, 116*(1), 132–152.

Weinberg, R. (2015). *The risk of a lifetime: How, when, and why procreation may be permissible.* Oxford University Press.

Wilkinson, S. (2010). *Choosing tomorrow's children.* Oxford University Press.

Williams, B. (1985). *Ethics and the limits of philosophy.* Harvard University Press.

Woodward, J. (1986). The non-identity problem. *Ethics, 96*(4), 804–831.

Conclusions

In this book, I explored how the boundaries of procreative responsibility are being redefined in light of the continuous development of Assisted Reproductive Technologies (ARTs), stemming from a person-affecting perspective.

In Chapter 1, I presented the currently available ARTs and prenatal treatments, such as *In Vitro* Fertilization (IVF), Preimplantation Genetic Diagnosis (PGD), prenatal genetic tests, carrier genetic testing, fetal therapy, and Mitochondrial Replacement Therapy (MRT). Furthermore, I introduced potential future ARTs, including *In Vitro* Gametogenesis (IVG), reproductive Genome Editing (rGE), and ectogenesis. I then acknowledged that, for many people, even before raising moral questions concerning procreative responsibility, ARTs raise ethical issues regarding their very permissibility and the consequences of their implementation. Since such issues would fall outside the purposes of the book, I considered the aforementioned ARTs effective tools available to prospective parents and thus legal, accessible, cheap, and morally legitimate. I also assumed that early embryos and fetuses do not have an intrinsic moral status. Finally, thanks to the conceptual tool of Pragmatic Optimism, I made another fundamental assumption regarding the greater accuracy and effectiveness of the currently available ARTs and the future possibility of IVG, rGE, and ectogenesis, as well as enhancement via genetic engineering.

In Chapter 2, I discussed some preliminary and crucial elements to understand and analyze procreative responsibility and the related principles or models proposed in the literature. First, I analyzed the general concept of responsibility, arguing that it can have at least six different meanings: virtue responsibility, role responsibility, outcome responsibility, causal responsibility, capacity responsibility, and liability responsibility. For the purposes of this book, I argued that the attribution of outcome responsibility to an agent depends on causal responsibility and the obligations the agent has toward others because of their specific role, or role responsibility, which in turn depends on the agent's moral, epistemic, and material capacities.

DOI: 10.4324/9781032654683-9

From this perspective, I maintained that an agent's material capabilities depend on external factors such as technological conditions. Therefore, I claimed that technological development increases human control over events that previously belonged to the domain of nature, and this generally extends human moral obligations toward others. I then discussed this argument in relation to the procreative context, suggesting that there is reason in favor of the argument that the continuous development of ARTs could inaugurate what has been defined as a colonization of reproduction by ethics. In light of this, I provided a formal definition of the concept of procreative responsibility, which is essential for a more comprehensive understanding of the various models proposed in the literature. I suggested that terms such as parental responsibility, procreative responsibility, and reproductive responsibility should not be used interchangeably. I argued that procreative responsibility encompasses the moral duties of those who are about to generate a future person. Within procreative responsibility, I identified two different sets of obligations: procreative-parental responsibility, which refers to the moral obligations of a parent in the procreative context; and reproductive responsibility, which pertains to the set of moral duties a reproducer has toward third parties or, for some, toward the world in general. Within reproductive responsibility, I further distinguished three categories: parental-reproductive responsibility, which pertains to the moral obligations that an individual has toward their existing children; family-based reproductive responsibility, which concerns the moral duties an individual has toward their own family unit; broad reproductive responsibility, which involves duties toward society and the world at large. In addition, I provided a further distinction within the domain of reproductive responsibility between quality-oriented reproductive responsibility, which arises when prospective parents are faced with the decision to bring into the world a child with specific characteristics, and quantity-oriented reproductive responsibility, which involves decisions about limiting the number of children to prevent negative impacts on other existing children, family members, or society due to concerns about overpopulation. Given this taxonomy, I have subsequently argued that prescriptions of procreative responsibility should not be understood as absolute moral duties or obligations but rather as *prima facie* ones; therefore, they should be balanced with other morally relevant aspects in the procreative context.

In the final part of Chapter 2, I argued that moral obligations falling within the sphere of procreative responsibility can depend not only on the development of ARTs but also on the definition of disability that prospective parents accept. Therefore, I analyzed four definitions of disability, first presenting the Social and the Medical models, considering them inappropriate to define this concept. Then, I presented the Welfarist and Equal

Opportunity models, claiming, without taking a definitive position between them, that these are more appropriate tools. These models consider disability as a social product but consider ARTs as legitimate tools to address disability. Reflection on disability served to define the notion of harm in the procreative context discussed in Chapter 4.

The remaining part of this book consisted of a philosophical analysis of the moral duties of future parents in the procreative context. I analyzed and criticized the most relevant procreative responsibility principles or models already discussed in the literature, and proposed new ones.

In Chapter 3, I discussed one of the most famous and influential procreative responsibility principles: the Principle of Procreative Beneficence (PPB). First, I presented its main characteristics, namely, its comparative and maximizing features and the *prima facie* nature of the moral obligations PPB prescribes. I then claimed that PPB may be criticized from both an internal and external perspective. Whereas the former challenges the principle *per se*, the latter challenges PPB based on its prescriptive scope in light of the complex balancing of person-affecting and impersonal reasons. With regard to the internal criticisms of PPB, I discussed several critiques, without claiming to exhaustively support or reject them. These include the eugenic criticism, the expressivist criticism, the criticism of internal normativity, the criticism of the comparative characteristic, the criticism of the concept of a better life, and the criticism of the neutrality of the definition of well-being. Then, I observed that PPB has a fourth feature that raises the most relevant problems from an internal perspective: PPB is also an impersonal model. Therefore, to explain this feature, I presented the Non-Identity Problem and some strategies trying to resolve this problem, including the *de dicto/de re* distinction and, most notably, the controversial perspective of impersonal harm in the maximizing and consequentialist terms defended by, among others, the utilitarian approach. Subsequently, I acknowledged that PPB adopts the same concept of impersonal harm defended by total utilitarianism. Thus, I stated that PPB is committed to accepting the Repugnant Conclusion, or at least a moral duty to reproduce, and that this provided further good reasons to reject such a model.

Despite the criticisms arising from the impersonal feature of PPB, I claimed that PPB is only weakly impersonal, as its proponents regard the obligations prescribes by the model as less binding than those involving the avoidance of personal harm to an actual person. This perspective allowed me to discuss the external criticisms of PPB, leading to the conclusion that PPB proponents are forced to acknowledge that the principle has very limited prescriptive force, even more so than they would be willing to accept. PPB loses its normative strength since it applies only when prospective parents already want to follow its prescriptions, or when they have no preference regarding which embryo to transfer *in utero*. In other words, PPB proponents do not provide any reasons for complying with the model's prescription rather than satisfying prospective parents' desires.

Given the problems associated with the notion of impersonal harm and the impersonal consequentialist and maximizing perspectives to procreation, in Chapter 4, I presented and assumed the consequences-based person-affecting morality as a robust starting point to discuss procreative duties that can be accepted from different moral perspectives. This approach considers solely person-affecting reasons dealing with procreative obligations and focuses on consequences, considering only the effects of actions and omissions, disregarding factors such as the agent's intentions.

From this perspecitve, I provided a discussion mainly focused on procreative-parental responsibility. I first presented the Minimum Threshold Model (MTM), and I discussed and rejected the criticism according to which the consequences-based person-affecting approach would not be able to justify the minimum moral duty that this model provides us with, namely, that it is morally wrong to procreate lives not worth living. Therefore, I claimed that MTM is an appropriate tool to guide procreative-parental choices in the context of selective ARTs, such as PGD.

I then considered the future availability of rGE. I argued that this technique is a non-identity-affecting practice, since rGE is employed on the embryo that shares numerical identity with the future individual. In this context, I proposed the Greater Moral Obligation View, namely, the thesis according to which the availability of rGE, in light of its non-identity-affecting nature, generates new moral obligations toward progeny, even accepting the very minimal constraints on procreative freedom in the field of selective reproductive techniques proposed by MTM. As a matter of fact, given the future availability of rGE, MTM will be an inappropriate model in informing procreative-parental choices. In this regard, I presented and discussed two original models of procreative-parental responsibility: the Bold Restriction of Procreative Autonomy and the Mild Restriction of Procreative Autonomy.

I argued that from a consequences-based person-affecting perspective, the Greater Moral Obligation View implies the Mild Restriction of Procreative Autonomy, arguing that only procreators who are already in the IVF process have a *prima facie* moral duty to transfer an embryo free from genetic diseases that meet the following criteria: (a) they are such diseases that are compatible with a life worth living, but they impair the child's psychological and physical well-being and/or significantly curtail the reasonable range of opportunities for choosing her own life plan; and (b) they are diseases for which, at the moment of IVF, safe treatment with rGE is available and legal, and it is not possible to treat them effectively *in vivo*.

I then applied these arguments to other non-identity-affecting techniques. I argued that prospective parents who employ IVG must grapple with the same obligations provided by the Mild Restriction of Procreative Autonomy. Although the Mild Restriction of Procreative Autonomy is a procreative-parental responsibility model that specifically relates to rGE, I argued that similar obligations should also be extended to MRT – as long as it involves pronuclear transfer – *in vivo* somatic gene therapy, and fetal therapy. Regarding the latter, I slightly modified the aforementioned formulation of the Mild Restriction of Procreative Autonomy, claiming that prospective parents have a moral duty to treat embryos or fetuses with diseases or conditions that meet the already mentioned criterion (a) and criterion (b)*, namely, conditions for which a safe and effective cure has been discovered at the time of pregnancy using the techniques in question, and it is not possible to cure them more or at least equally effectively after the child's birth. I also considered both partial and total ectogenesis, arguing that although this technology cannot be directly described as a non-identity-affecting technique, it would make it possible to have the ideal place to apply interventions through aforementioned non-identity-affecting ARTs. Therefore, I argued that regarding complete ectogenesis, there may be a *prima facie* moral duty to resort to it in order to avoid conditions that meet the criteria discussed above only for prospective parents who are already in the IVF process. With regard to partial ectogenesis, which allows the viability of the fetus several weeks before birth, I claimed in this context that moral reasons would emerge to transfer the fetus already in the mother's uterus into the artificial womb for as long as possible to guarantee the future child any treatments that meet the criteria mentioned above.

Toward the end of Chapter 4, I argued that to provide a more comprehensive account of procreative responsibility, the outlined prescriptions of procreative-parental responsibility should be integrated with others, namely, the reproductive responsibility prescriptions. In this context, I presented two models of this kind that are compatible with the consequences-based person-affecting morality: Procreative Altruism – renamed Reproductive Altruism – and the Principle of Generalized Procreative Non-Maleficence – renamed the Principle of Generalized Reproductive Non-Maleficence. I argued that both models can offer additional reasons to avoid harm or promote the well-being of third parties through reproductive choice. I then pointed out that, since I focus more on procreative-parental responsibility in the book, these reasons should be further evaluated in the debate.

In Chapter 5, I acknowledged that the Greater Moral Obligation View relies on the fundamental but controversial claim that rGE is a non-identity-affecting procedure. Then, I conceptualized and rejected four objections to this assumption. I first discussed the identity objection, according to which, due to the modification via rGE, the embryo will develop into a person who is numerically different from the one who would have developed had the modification not occurred. I argued that the extent and the implications of this critique depend on the metaphysical assumption regarding identity. Hence, I presented four versions of this critique, which consider, respectively, the identity (i) as the persistence of the genetic material, (ii) as an integrated whole, (iii) as psychological continuity, and (iv) as an organism. After questioning some implications of its stronger formulations, I argued that the identity objection is more effective the more significant the modification's magnitude and effects are. However, I claimed that this does not provide a conclusive reason for rejecting the non-identity-affecting assumption. Furthermore, I claimed that if a biologist account of identity is assumed and, at the same time, we maintain that the zygote already has a well-established identity, then it can even be concluded that almost all modifications via rGE – even the most disruptive ones – do not change the numerical identity.

I then discussed the critique of the necessity of rGE for the existence of the modified individual, which states that whenever prospective parents decide to undergo the IVF process in order to use rGE, the resulting child cannot be benefited or harmed by this decision, since the choice to undergo rGE determines their identity. I replied that our moral duties depend on the context in which we act. Considering this, I observed a moral difference between the pre- and post-conception scenarios. Unlike the former, in the latter, there is an early embryo that is numerically identical to the future individual. I claimed that treating – or not treating – this embryo with rGE at this moment does not determine the identity of the future child but may affect a specific future person. Therefore, it is morally irrelevant that the embryo was created only to be treated.

I then addressed the "artificially constrained future" objection, which states that the non-identity-affecting assumption holds only in rare cases where the modified child would have been brought into existence even if rGE had not been employed. Here, the morally relevant counterfactuals to assess whether the modification harms or benefits the future child concern the will of the parents if rGE is not available. I argued that this objection failed to be effective because it confuses two morally distinct propositions: (a) the child could not have existed in a condition other than that in which they find themself; and (b) the prospective parents did not want the child to exist in a different condition than the one in which they are. Because of this confusion, there is a moral short circuit, according to which counterfactual scenarios should be compared to assess whether the future child has experienced harm or benefit and, consequently, the morality of the parent's conduct, but it seems that the counterfactual scenarios to be compared are voluntarily decided by the same people who carry out the action under moral scrutiny. I rejected this position, arguing that the moral relevance of counterfactuals for evaluating the occurrence of a harm or a benefit to a future child depends both on the actual conditions of the child's existence in the various alternative scenarios and the material capabilities of the prospective parents, who through their actions or omissions can actualize a scenario over another in which the future child may be harmed or benefited.

I finally addressed the critique of the inevitability of PGD, according to which rGE will likely involve the creation and modification of more embryos, followed by the selection of the embryo(s) to be transferred via PGD. Therefore, rGE cannot yet be considered purely non-identity-affecting since selection via PGD is inevitable. However, I argued that to evaluate new moral obligations to offspring, we must focus not on the reproductive process but on the resulting child. I observed that regardless of the need for PGD after rGE, the resulting child would, in any case, have been in a position to be benefited or harmed by rGE and, therefore, would have good reasons to complain against the parents if harmed. I then concluded that rGE can be reasonably considered a non-identity-affecting technique and, as a consequence, the new moral duties within the sphere of procreative-parental responsibility proposed in Chapter 4 are legitimate.

In Chapter 6, I acknowledged that Mild Restriction of Procreative Autonomy, which I defended in the previous chapters, primarily aims to determine the *circumstances* in which moral duties toward the future child emerge and not so much to specify exhaustively the *contents* of such duties. I thus claimed that the purpose of this model was to find a first common ground that can be shared by different moral perspectives, which however recognize in the person-affecting perspective moral reasons to inform procreators conduct. Nonetheless, as a negative model, I acknowledged that the Mild Restriction of Procreative Autonomy does not exhaust moral reflection on what prospective parents should do from a procreative-parental perspective. Therefore, I investigated whether the Greater Moral Obligation View implies that future parents who are already in the IVF process are morally obliged not only to avoid harm to future children but also to enhance their future children through rGE. Without claiming completeness, I analyzed this issue through the lens of the Child's Right to an Open Future (CROF) argument. From this perspective, I first argued that CROF is not in conflict with genetic enhancements that do not constrain the child to a life project decided by the parents, thus limiting the development of their autonomy. Genetic enhancements such as expanding the future individual's lifespan, improving human vision, or even enhancing memory or general intelligence in some cases might not be considered in conflict with CROF. However, I acknowledged that it would be reasonable to delay enhancement interventions until a person reaches maturity to decide for themselves, except for the interventions mentioned above that should be performed very early in life to have the desired effect. I also stated that CROF does not entail that parents have any moral obligation to open as many options as possible for their children; rather, they should provide them with a reasonable range of opportunities. I observed that this depends on the dominant cooperative framework, which however can change over time. Therefore, I claimed that the moral obligations predicted by CROF change as the dominant cooperative scheme changes.

In light of this, I concluded that, based on CROF, the Greater Moral Obligation View entails that in the current dominant cooperative scheme, prospective parents are not morally obligated to genetically enhance their children, as an unenhanced person possessing traits in line with the normal functioning of the species already has access to a reasonable range of opportunities. However, if the dominant cooperative framework were to change, requiring cognitive and physical capacities only achievable through genetic enhancement, parents would be morally obliged to use such practices to provide their children with a reasonable range of opportunities.

Chapters 3–6 discussed procreative responsibility primarily focusing on the consequences of future parents' choices. In Chapter 7, assuming that, in addition to harms and benefits to actual people, intentions and attitudes can also play a role in moral judgment for many people, I investigated the moral relevance of these aspects in ARTs in a way compatible with person-affecting morality. As in Chapter 4, I addressed selective techniques first, followed by non-identity-affecting ones. I initially presented the parental virtue approach, arguing that it does not offer reasons why the parental virtues of acceptingness, parental commitment, and the future-agent-focus should also be extended in the procreative realm. I then presented two proposals which, although starting from distinct moral assumptions, attempt to justify the moral relevance of parental intentions and attitudes in the realm of procreation: the Principle of Deliberate Impossibility and – from a perspective of responsibility that is more reproductive than procreative-prarental – the collective interests account.

In light of the inadequacy of the first and the partiality of the second, I proposed a new argument that emphasizes the importance of the parent-child relationship. I called this the Parent – Child Relationship argument. It suggests that procreative decisions imply two desires: the desire to create a child – not subject to moral blame – and the desire that the embryo develops under a specific condition, which is a person-affecting attitude and is morally relevant to determining our procreative obligations. From this perspective, I argued that procreating via IVF plus PGD can be morally problematic in some circumstances, even if it does not directly harm anyone. Furthermore, I argued that selecting embryos for non-health-related traits, such as eye color or sex, does not necessarily conflict with the Parent–Child Relationship argument.

Then, and most importantly, I applied the Parent–Child Relationship argument to a scenario where rGE and complete ectogenesis are available. In this context, I argued that employing such techniques may not only be in line with the promotion of the parent–child relationship but may also enhance it, showing a greater propensity by parents to take care of their children's interests and protect them. Support for this comes from the fact that prospective parents' second implicit desire in deciding to parent a child is for that child to develop in a place – whether *in vitro* or in an artificial womb – where it is easier to be protected from a condition of suffering or disability. Therefore, I argued that the Greater Moral Obligation View demands more than what the Mild Restriction of Procreative Autonomy requires. In light of this, I claimed that the Bold Restriction of Procreative Autonomy should be rehabilitated: given the technological and economic possibility to do so, *all* prospective parents would have moral reasons to reproduce through IVF plus rGE if needed or ectogenesis, as through such practices the parental attitudes of care and protection required of the future parent would be more extensively valued and promoted.

Finally, I returned to the previous accounts dealing with procreative intentions and attitudes, stating that the argument in support of the Bold Restriction of Procreative Autonomy is not defensible only through the Parent–Child Relationship argument. On the contrary, all the other accounts presented above support the idea that the availability of rGE and ectogenesis, as practices that extend control over the traits of future children, raise moral reasons to prefer artificial reproduction to natural reproduction.

These conclusions represent the outcome of a still ongoing reflection within the field of responsibility and reproduction. Much work remains to be done to deepen issues I discussed, only mentioned, or even not considered in these pages. As a general remark, many questions remain open. Precisely because of the desire to propose theses that different moral perspectives could share, I often avoided taking a specific position on some issues, such as the concept of harm and the more appropriate definition of disability. Moreover, since I mainly focused on procreative-parental responsibility, further discussion is needed concerning reproductive responsibility and how these two components of procreative responsibility should be balanced to provide a comprehensive and more general account. Addressing these issues is undoubtedly necessary to further develop research in this area.

Notwithstanding that, I believe this book provides strong arguments in support of the Greater Moral Obligation View, according to which, in light of the future availability of non-identity-affecting ARTs – particularly rGE and ectogenesis – prospective parents will face a greater moral obligation toward their offspring compared to obligations faced in a context where only current, identity-affecting ARTs are available. This will significantly extend the boundaries of procreative-parental responsibility and, consequently, procreative responsibility. This thesis appears to be broadly supported across various moral perspectives, which acknowledge the moral relevance of consequences-based person-affecting, and/or intentions and attitudes in a way compatible with person-affecting morality.

The claim in favor of an extension of procreative responsibility in light of the continuous development of ARTs is undoubtedly not a new argument in the debate and, as I argued throughout this work, others before me have supported it. However, the originality of my proposal lies precisely in the specific kind of defense that I proposed and in the theoretical assumptions I have made. Generally, person-affecting morality has been mainly used in the selective context to support substantial procreative freedom, like that proposed by MTM, and not to assert new moral obligations. On the contrary, I hope to have shown that even stemming from this theoretical background, in light of the future availability of non-identity-affecting ARTs, we are still committed to supporting the existence of greater moral obligations for prospective parents toward their offspring. However, such greater moral obligations do not naively provide definitive solutions; the philosophical-rational tools employed, while fundamental, cannot fully capture the extreme complexity and intricacy of human reproduction, nor can they offer definitive guidance on how to act in such contexts. Therefore, this book is a modest attempt to understand the moral reasons at stake: an attempt aimed not so much at a complete understanding, but at least a deeper one than that which does not go beyond the intuitions that inevitably each of us possesses when discussing topics described in this work. While not providing definitive answers, this book offers *reasons* that should at least be considered in the procreative context and which – I hope – will be able to inform the choices of the procreators of tomorrow.

There are more things in heaven and earth, Horatio, than are dreamt of in your philosophy.

W. Shakespeare, Hamlet I, V

Acknowledgments

The book *Procreative Responsibility and Assisted Reproductive Technologies* is an expansion and development of my doctoral thesis in Clinical and Experimental Medicine and Medical Humanities, which I defended at the University of Insubria in December 2021. After further elaboration during my research period at the IRCCS San Raffaele Hospital Scientific Institute, the thesis was translated, updated, and substantially revised into this book at the University of Bergamo, where I am currently a postdoctoral researcher. This final version has also undoubtedly benefited from my teaching activities in Bioethics since 2021 within the Politics, Philosophy, and Public Affairs program at the University of Milan and Vita-Salute San Raffaele University, Milan. I am grateful to these institutions for providing a great environment and academic freedom for my research. In this regard, I would like to thank Giorgio Casari, Corrado Del Bò, Mario Picozzi, and Massimo Reichlin. My research was significantly supported also by stays at various institutions, including the Centre for Biomedical Ethics and Law at KU Leuven, the Ethox Centre (University of Oxford), and especially the Uehiro Centre for Practical Ethics (University of Oxford), which hosted me during my research path. I am deeply thankful to these centers for their hospitality and the stimulating academic environment they provided.

In addition, the book revisits and expands, sometimes using the same wording, the content from three papers – two published by *Bioethics* in 2023 and 2021 and one published by *Phenomenology and Mind* in 2020. I thank these journals for allowing me to reuse the material, which is essential for a comprehensive view of my thoughts on the topics addressed. Moreover, I am grateful to Routledge, in particular to Rosaleah Stammler and Andrew Weckenmann, for the decision to publish this book and for the great availability and kindness shown in the writing process.

In these early years of my academic career, I have come to profoundly understand that research is a collective effort, even when only one name appears on the covers of books. The considerations in this work are the result of experiences, meetings, and passionate discussions with extraordinary

232 *Acknowledgments*

people. Thanks to them, I have been able to grow, refine, and revise my ideas, leading to the present version of this work. In addition to the scholars I have mentioned before, I would like to thank Giacomo Maria Arrigo, Elvio Baccarini, Andrew Barnhart, Federico Bina, Simone Bondesan, Pascal Borry, Emma Capulli, Giulia Cavaliere, Alice Cavolo, Francesca Cerea, Silvia Ceruti, Francesca Cesarano, Ben Davis, Elena Ferioli, Alessandra Gasparetto, Alberto Giubilini, Alessandra Grossi, Sergio Filippo Magni, Luca Marelli, Mario Marotta, Simone Marsilio, Carlo Martini, Roberto Mordacci, Federico Nicoli, César Palacios-González, Giulio Pennacchioni, Federico Pennestrì, Stefano Pinzan, Virginia Sanchini, Sara Roggi, Roberta Sala, Sarah Songorian, Luigi Scollo, Luca Stroppa, and Alessandro Volpe. Special thanks to Silvia Camporesi, Paola Carrera, Tess Johnson, and Gary O'Brien, who carefully read and commented on the first drafts of my book, which would certainly have been worse without their help.

Further special thanks to Massimo Reichlin, from whom I hope I have managed to absorb at least a fraction of his philosophical rigor and research skills. I owe him a great debt for his invaluable contribution to my academic development, for meticulously reviewing most of my works, including this book, and for always helping me refine and clarify my thoughts.

Finally, I would like to express my deepest gratitude to Giada, Irene, Bruno, and Nicolò, who have supported me most patiently, even during the most challenging times.

Index

For Product Safety Concerns and Information please contact our EU
representative GPSR@taylorandfrancis.com
Taylor & Francis Verlag GmbH, Kaufingerstraße 24, 80331 München, Germany

www.ingramcontent.com/pod-product-compliance
Lightning Source LLC
Chambersburg PA
CBHW060253220326
41598CB00027B/4088